Retinopathy of Prematurity

Editors

GRAHAM E. QUINN
ALISTAIR R. FIELDER

CLINICS IN PERINATOLOGY

www.perinatology.theclinics.com

Consulting Editor
LUCKY JAIN

June 2013 • Volume 40 • Number 2

ELSEVIER

1600 John F. Kennedy Boulevard • Suite 1800 • Philadelphia, Pennsylvania, 19103-2899

http://www.theclinics.com

CLINICS IN PERINATOLOGY Volume 40, Number 2
June 2013 ISSN 0095-5108, ISBN-13: 978-1-4557-7137-0

Editor: Kerry Holland
Developmental Editor: Donald Mumford

Clinics in Perinatology (ISSN 0095-5108) is published quarterly by Elsevier Inc., 360 Park Avenue South, New York, NY 10010-1710. Months of issue are March, June, September, and December. Business and Editorial Offices: 1600 John F. Kennedy Blvd., Ste. 1800, Philadelphia, PA 19103-2899. Customer Service Office: 3251 Riverport Lane, Maryland Heights, MO 63043. Periodicals postage paid at New York, NY and additional mailing offices. Subscription prices are $273.00 per year (US individuals), $401.00 per year (US institutions), $326.00 per year (Canadian individuals), $509.00 per year (Canadian institutions), $400.00 per year (foreign individuals), $509.00 per year (foreign institutions), $129.00 per year (US students), and $186.00 per year (Canadian and foreign students). Foreign air speed delivery is included in all Clinics subscription prices. All prices are subject to change without notice. **POSTMASTER:** Send address changes to *Clinics in Perinatology*, Elsevier Health Sciences Division, Subscription Customer Service, 3251 Riverport Lane, Maryland Heights, MO 63043. **Customer Service: Telephone: 1-800-654-2452** (U.S. and Canada); **1-314-447-8871** (outside U.S. and Canada). **Fax: 1-314-447-8029. E-mail: journalscustomerservice-usa@elsevier.com** (for print support); **journalsonlinesupport-usa@elsevier.com** (for online support).

Reprints. For copies of 100 or more, of articles in this publication, please contact the Commercial Reprints Department, Elsevier Inc., 360 Park Avenue South, New York, NY 10010-1710. Tel. (212) 633-3812; Fax: (212) 482-1935; E-mail: reprints@elsevier.com.

Clinics in Perinatology is also published in Spanish by McGraw-Hill Interamericana Editores S.A., P.O. Box 5-237, 06500 Mexico D.F., Mexico.

Clinics in Perinatology is covered in *MEDLINE/PubMed (Index Medicus) Current Contents, Excepta Medica, BIOSIS and ISI/BIOMED.*

Printed and bound by CPI Group (UK) Ltd, Croydon, CR0 4YY

Transferred to digital print 2012

Contributors

CONSULTING EDITOR

LUCKY JAIN, MD, MBA
Richard W. Blumberg Professor and Executive Vice Chairman, Department of Pediatrics;
Medical Director, Emory Children's Center, Emory University School of Medicine, Atlanta,
Georgia

EDITORS

GRAHAM E. QUINN, MD, MSCE
Professor of Ophthalmology, Division of Ophthalmology, The Children's Hospital of
Philadelphia, University of Pennsylvania Perelman School of Medicine, Philadelphia,
Pennsylvania

ALISTAIR R. FIELDER, FRCP, FRCS, FRCOphth
Professor Emeritus of Ophthalmology, Department of Optometry and Visual Science,
City University, London, United Kingdom

AUTHORS

RAJVARDHAN AZAD, MBBS, MD, FRCSed
Chief and Professor, Dr. R.P. Centre for Ophthalmic Sciences, All India Institute of Medical
Sciences, New Delhi, India

GIL BINENBAUM, MD, MSCE
Division of Ophthalmology, The Children's Hospital of Philadelphia, Philadelphia,
Pennsylvania

BRIAN A. DARLOW, MD, FRCP, FRACP, FRCPCH
Cure Kids Professor of Paediatric Research, Department of Paediatrics, University
of Otago Christchurch, Christchurch, New Zealand

ANNA L. ELLS, MD, FRCS(C)
Department of Ophthalmology, University of Calgary, Alberta, Canada

ALISTAIR R. FIELDER, FRCP, FRCS, FRCOphth
Professor Emeritus of Ophthalmology, Department of Optometry and Visual Science,
City University, London, United Kingdom

BRIAN W. FLECK, MD, FRCOph
Consultant Ophthalmologist, Department of Ophthalmology, Princess Alexandra
Eye Pavilion, Edinburgh, United Kingdom

CLARE E. GILBERT, MD, MSc, FRCOphth
Professor of International Eye Health, Department of Clinical Research, London School
of Hygiene and Tropical Medicine, London, United Kingdom

GLEN A. GOLE, MD BS (NSW), FRANZCO, FRACS
Professor of Ophthalmology, Discipline of Paediatrics and Child Health, The Royal
Children's Hospital, The University of Queensland, Brisbane, Queensland, Australia

ANNA-LENA HARD, MD, PhD
Section of Pediatric Ophthalmology, The Queen Silvia Children's Hospital, The
Sahlgrenska Academy at University of Gothenburg, Göteborg, Sweden

ANN HELLSTRÖM, MD, PhD
Professor of Ophthalmology, Section of Pediatric Ophthalmology, The Queen Silvia
Children's Hospital, The Sahlgrenska Academy at University of Gothenburg, Göteborg,
Sweden

GERD HOLMSTRÖM, MD, PhD
Professor, Department of Neuroscience/Ophthalmology, University Hospital, Uppsala
University, Uppsala, Sweden

EVA LARSSON, MD, PhD
Associate Professor, Department of Neuroscience/Ophthalmology, University Hospital,
Uppsala University, Uppsala, Sweden

RAMIRO S. MALDONADO, MD
Department of Ophthalmology, Duke University Medical Center, Durham, North Carolina

GRAHAM E. QUINN, MD, MSCE
Professor of Ophthalmology, Division of Ophthalmology, The Children's Hospital of
Philadelphia, University of Pennsylvania Perelman School of Medicine, Philadelphia,
Pennsylvania

ANA M. QUIROGA, RN, BSN
Professor of Neonatal Nursing, School of Nursing, Universidad Austral, Buenos Aires;
Argentina and National Program of Infant Blindness Prevention due to Retinopathy of
Prematurity, National Ministry of Health, Argentina

LOIS E. SMITH, MD, PhD
Professor of Ophthalmology, Department of Ophthalmology, Children's Hospital Boston,
Harvard Medical School, Boston, Massachusetts

BEN J. STENSON, MD
Consultant Neonatologist, Neonatal Unit, Simpson Centre for Reproductive Health, Royal
Infirmary of Edinburgh, Edinburgh, United Kingdom

CYNTHIA A. TOTH, MD
Department of Ophthalmology, Duke University Medical Center; Department of Biomedical
Engineering, Pratt School of Engineering, Duke University, Durham, North Carolina

DAVID K. WALLACE, MD, MPH
Professor of Ophthalmology and Pediatrics, Director of Clinical Research, Department
of Ophthalmology and Pediatrics, Duke Eye Center, Durham, North Carolina

CLARE M. WILSON, MRCOphth, PhD
Department of Visual Neuroscience, UCL Institute of Ophthalmology, London, United
Kingdom

KATHERINE Y. WU, BS
Department of Ophthalmology and Pediatrics, Duke Eye Center; Duke University School
of Medicine, Durham, North Carolina

PEIQUAN ZHAO, MD
Professor, Xinhua Hospital, School of Medicine, Shanghai Jiao Tong University,
Shanghai, China

ANDREA ZIN, MD, MSc, PhD
Research Associate, Clinical Research Unit, Fernandes Figueira Institute, Flamengo,
Rio de Janeiro, Brazil

Contents

Retinopathy of prematurity (ROP) in high-income countries now occurs, mostly in extreme low birth weight infants. In those countries, the incidence of ROP seems to have declined incrementally over the last few decades. But in middle-income countries, high rates of premature birth and increasing resuscitation of premature infants, often with suboptimal standards of care, have resulted in a third epidemic of ROP. Improved maternal and neonatal care, ROP screening guidelines appropriate for middle-income countries, and widespread timely treatment are urgently called for to control this third epidemic.

Retinopathy of prematurity occurs because the retina of a preterm infant at birth is incompletely vascularized, and if the postnatal environment does not match the in utero environment that supported retinal development, the vessels and neural retina will not grow normally. Risk factors determined from many clinical studies and animal studies fall into 2 categories: prenatal factors and postnatal factors.

Retinopathy of prematurity (ROP) programs require collaboration between neonatologists, ophthalmologists, nurses, and allied health personnel, together with parents. The concept of a ROP program will vary according to the setting. However, in every situation there should be 2 main aspects: primary prevention of ROP through better overall care, and secondary prevention through case detection (often called screening), treatment, and follow-up. ROP programs will have different content and emphasis according to whether the setting is in an economically advanced or developing country.

with ROP. Finally, we explore how this novel information may affect our understanding of ROP and the possible implications in vision and retinal development.

David K. Wallace and Katherine Y. Wu

Treatment for retinopathy of prematurity (ROP) is indicated when type 1 disease is present. The Early Treatment for Retinopathy of Prematurity (ETROP) clinical trial established that laser treatment of severe ROP has a high rate of visual and anatomic success. Recently, anti–vascular endothelial growth factor (VEGF) drugs such as bevacizumab have been used in lieu of or in addition to laser treatment. Results are promising, but long-term outcomes and systemic side effects are unknown. Future studies are needed to determine whether anti-VEGF treatment is superior to laser and, if so, which drug and dose are safe and effective.

Gerd Holmström and Eva Larsson

In prematurely born children, various visual and ophthalmologic sequelae occur because of both retinopathy of prematurity (ROP) and preterm birth per se. Several long-term follow-up studies have described the outcome of ROP. Visual impairment and blindness are well-known consequences, but the prevalence varies globally because of differing neonatal and ophthalmologic care. Improving treatment options and criteria for the treatment of ROP are continuously changing the ophthalmologic outcome. The anatomic outcome has improved with treatment, but good anatomic outcome in treated severe ROP does not always reflect the functional outcome. There is no consensus regarding long-term follow-up of prematurely born children.

Graham E. Quinn, Alistair R. Fielder, Rajvardhan Azad, and Peiquan Zhao

The third World Retinopathy of Prematurity (ROP) Congress, held in Shanghai in October 2012, showed that international collaborations have already built up from the previous 2 events. The participants learned about ROP from across the world: who it affects and its behavior, and in a way that would not be possible from the literature. Emerging technologies and treatments are set to have a major impact on the identification and treatment of ROP. Undoubtedly, the picture will have changed dramatically by the fourth World ROP Congress in Mexico in 3 years.

PROGRAM OBJECTIVE

The goal of *Clinics in Perinatology* is to keep practicing perinatologists, neonatologists, obstetricians, practicing physicians and residents up to date with current clinical practice in perinatology by providing timely articles reviewing the state of the art in patient care.

TARGET AUDIENCE

Perinatologists, neonatologists, obstetricians, practicing physicians, residents and healthcare professionals who provide patient care utilizing findings from *Clinics in Perinatology*.

LEARNING OBJECTIVES

Upon completion of this activity, participants will be able to:

1. Review lessons learned from recent randomized trials in regards to retinopathy of prematurity and the oxygen conundrum.
2. Discuss setting up and improving retinopathy of prematurity programs to include the interaction of neonatology, nursing and ophthalmology.
3. Recognize the current and future trends in treatment of severe retinopathy of prematurity.

ACCREDITATION

The Elsevier Office of Continuing Medical Education (EOCME) is accredited by the Accreditation Council for Continuing Medical Education (ACCME) to provide continuing medical education for physicians.

The EOCME designates this enduring material for a maximum of 15 *AMA PRA Category 1 Credit*(s)™. Physicians should claim only the credit commensurate with the extent of their participation in the activity.

All other health care professionals requesting continuing education credit for this enduring material will be issued a certificate of participation.

DISCLOSURE OF CONFLICTS OF INTEREST

The EOCME assesses conflict of interest with its instructors, faculty, planners, and other individuals who are in a position to control the content of CME activities. All relevant conflicts of interest that are identified are thoroughly vetted by EOCME for fair balance, scientific objectivity, and patient care recommendations. EOCME is committed to providing its learners with CME activities that promote improvements or quality in healthcare and not a specific proprietary business or a commercial interest.

The planning committee, staff, authors and editors listed below have identified no financial relationships or relationships to products or devices they or their spouse/life partner have with commercial interest related to the content of this CME activity:

Rajvardhan Azad, MBBS, MD, FRCSed; Gil Binenbaum, MD, MSCE; Nicole Congleton; Brian Darlow, MA,MB, BChir MD (Cantab), FRCP, FRCPCH; Brian Fleck, MD, FRCOphth, FRCS; Clare E. Gilbert, MD, MSc, FRCOphth; Glen Gole, MB BS (NSW), MD (NSW), FRANZCO, FRACS; Anna-Lena Hard, MD, PhD; Ann Hellstrom, MD, PhD; Kerry Holland; Gerd Holmstrom, MD; Lucky Jain, MD, MBA; Eva Larsson, MD; Sandy Lavery; Ramiro S. Maldonado, MD; Jill McNair; Palani Murugesan; Graham E. Quinn, MD, MSCE; Ana Quiroga, RN, BSN; Lois Smith, MD, PhD; Ben Stenson, MD, FRCPCH; David Wallace, MD, MPH; Katherine Wu, BS; Peiquan Zhao, MD; and Andrea Zin, MD, MSc.

The planning committee, staff, authors and editors listed below have identified financial relationships or relationships to products or devices they or their spouse/life partner have with commercial interest related to the content of this CME activity:

Anna L. Ells, MD, FRCS is a consultant/advisor for Clarity Systems, Inc. (Retcam).

Alistair Fielder, FRCP, FRCS, FRCOphth is on the speaker's bureau for Clarity Medical Systems and is a consultant/advisor for Novartis Pharma AG.

Cynthia Toth, MD has royalties/patents with Alcon Laboratories; research grant money from Bioptigen, Genentech, and Physical Sciences, Inc.

Claire Wilson, MRCOphth is a named inventor on patent held by UCL for image analysis software.

UNAPPROVED/OFF-LABEL USE DISCLOSURE

The EOCME requires CME faculty to disclose to the participants:

1. When products or procedures being discussed are off-label, unlabelled, experimental, and/or investigational (not US Food and Drug Administration (FDA) approved); and
2. Any limitations on the information presented, such as data that are preliminary or that represent ongoing research, interim analyses, and/or unsupported opinions. Faculty may discuss information about pharmaceutical agents that is outside of FDA-approved labelling. This information is intended solely for CME and is not intended to promote off-label use of these medications. If you have any questions, contact the medical affairs department of the manufacturer for the most recent prescribing information.

TO ENROLL

To enroll in the *Clinics in Perinatology* Continuing Medical Education program, call customer service at 1-800-654-2452 or sign up online at http://www.theclinics.com/home/cme. The CME program is available to subscribers for an additional annual fee of $212 USD.

METHOD OF PARTICIPATION

In order to claim credit, participants must complete the following:

1. Complete enrolment as indicated above.
2. Read the activity.
3. Complete the CME Test and Evaluation. Participants must achieve a score of 70% on the test. All CME Tests and Evaluations must be completed online.

CME INQUIRIES/SPECIAL NEEDS

For all CME inquiries or special needs, please contact elsevierCME@elsevier.com.

CLINICS IN PERINATOLOGY

RELATED INTEREST

Pediatric Clinics of North America, Volume 60, Issue 1 (February 2013)
Breastfeeding Updates for the Pediatrician
Ardythe Morrow, MD, and Caroline Chantry, MD, *Editors*

NOW AVAILABLE FOR YOUR iPhone and iPad

Foreword

The Intertwined Paths of Retinopathy of Prematurity and Neonatal Intensive Care

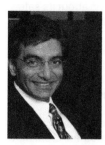

Lucky Jain, MD, MBA
Consulting Editor

The story of retinopathy of prematurity (ROP) and its evolution in the last 70 years is remarkably linked to the evolution of neonatal care itself.[1] From a sporadic disease affecting preterm infants in resource-rich countries, ROP now has now become a global disease. The growing success of neonatal care in less developed countries is enabling survival of tiny premature infants; it is also replaying the saga of ROP-related blindness from many decades ago.[2] Indeed, several remarkable features of this intertwined story deserve to be highlighted and are elegantly covered in this issue of the *Clinics in Perinatology*.

First, the disease highlights challenges clinicians face every day; actions designed to protect one organ system can have detrimental consequences on another. Inadequate oxygen delivery leads to death and lifelong disability; provision of too much supplemental oxygen, particularly in the absence of adequate controls and monitoring, leads to ROP and blindness.[2] As neonatal care evolves around the globe, neonatologists and ophthalmologists need to work diligently to prevent missteps of the past. There is also the conundrum of how much oxygen is too much and what oxygen saturation levels are ideal for premature infants.[3] It may well be that the biphasic nature of angiopathy requires lower saturation levels in early phases of the disease as compared to the later stages encountered in the more mature preterm infant.[4] However, research targeting saturation levels is fraught with logistical difficulties as exemplified by the Support Trial.[5] Another such trial which aimed at higher oxygen saturations failed to show a reduction in severity of ROP and had an added burden of worsening chronic lung disease.[6]

Second, even within countries with advanced neonatal care, the disease continues to evolve. Survival of neonates at the limits of viability is bringing new challenges. These neonates often have more complex presentations of ROP and have need for

Clin Perinatol 40 (2013) xiii–xv
http://dx.doi.org/10.1016/j.clp.2013.04.002
0095-5108/13/$ – see front matter © 2013 Published by Elsevier Inc.

perinatology.theclinics.com

repeated interventions with frequent transfers to tertiary care centers. Telemedicine can reduce some of these trips, but we need more reliable linkups and imaging techniques for us to reach a better level of comfort.

Third, basic science research is needed to further refine our understanding of mechanisms underlying retinal injury and repair. Angiogenesis is a complex process involving a series of growth factors, including the rate-limiting vascular endothelial growth factor (VEGF).[7] The discovery that VEGF can be targeted to reduce tumor growth has led to exciting applications of VEGF inhibitors in diseases such as ROP where excessive angiogenesis plays a major role. However, questions about its safety remain, and as authors in this *Clinics in Perinatology* point out, this therapy will need to be monitored closely before it can supplant laser therapy.

Finally, uniform guidelines for screening and management of premature infants for ROP have had enormous impact on reducing the incidence of disabling ROP. The most recent version of these guidelines for screening examination of preterm infants was published earlier this year and represents a remarkable ongoing collaboration between pediatricians, ophthalmologists, and optometrists.[8]

Overall, this issue of the *Clinics in Perinatology* brings together experts from various fields related to ROP. Drs Quinn and Fielder are to be congratulated for creating a remarkable resource of review articles with state-of-the-art information about this important disease. I am also grateful to Kerry Holland and Elsevier for their support and to readers everywhere who continue to further their quest for knowledge and better patient care.

Lucky Jain, MD, MBA
Department of Pediatrics
Emory Children's Center
Emory University School of Medicine
2015 Uppergate Drive
Atlanta, GA 30322, USA

E-mail address:
ljain@emory.edu

REFERENCES

1. Terry TL. Extreme prematurity and fibroblastic overgrowth of persistent vascular sheath behind each crystalline lens: 1. Preliminary report. Am J Ophthalmol 1942;25:203–4.

2. Ashton N, Ward B, Serpell G. Effect of oxygen on developing retinal vessels with particular reference to the problem of retrolental fibroplasias. Br J Ophthalmol 1954;38:397–432.

3. Cherian S, Morris I, Evans J, et al. Oxygen therapy in preterm infants. Paediatr Respir Rev 2013. http://dx.doi.org/10.1016/j.prrv.2012.12.003.

4. Martinelli S, Gatelli I, Proto A. SpO_2 and retinopathy of prematurity: state of the art. J Mat Fetal Med 2012;25:108–10.

5. SUPPORT Study Group of the Eunice Kennedy Shriver NICHD Neonatal Research Network. Target ranges of oxygen saturation in extremely preterm infants. N Engl J Med 2010;362:1959–69.

6. The STOP-ROP Multicenter Study Group. Supplemental therapeutic oxygen for prethreshold retinopathy of prematurity (STOP-ROP), a randomized, controlled trial. I: primary outcomes. Pediatrics 2000;105:295–310.

7. Hartnett ME, Penn JS. Mechanism and management of retinopathy of prematurity. N Engl J Med 2012;367:2515–26.
8. Fierson WM, American Academy of Pediatrics Section on Ophthalmology, American Academy of Ophthalmology, American Association for Pediatric Ophthalmology and Strabismus, American Association of Certified Orthoptists. Screening examination of premature infants for retinopathy of prematurity. Pediatrics 2013;131:189–95.

Preface

Prevention of ROP Blindness

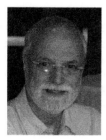
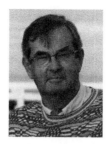

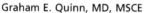

Graham E. Quinn, MD, MSCE   Alistair R. Fielder, FRCP, FRCS, FRCOphth
Editors

Blindness from retinopathy of prematurity (ROP) has become a disease no longer confined to the countries that developed neonatal intensive care units (NICUs) more than a half century ago; the vast majority of babies blinded from the disease are cared for in countries where the development of NICUs has become a logical extension of improving medical care.[1,2] This imposes a burden of blindness on societies that may have limited resources, both human and equipment, and that may, initially at least, have little awareness of the developing problem. The epidemiology of ROP blindness, with emphasis on recent regional changes and on regions that have epidemic proportions of ROP blindness, is highlighted by Zin and Gole in this issue. Also in this issue is a report of the recent World ROP Congress held in October 2012, which highlights the importance of international collaboration in prevention, detection, and treatment of serious ROP.

The challenges of identifying those babies at risk for ROP blindness are multifaceted and several of the articles included here address that complex issue. Since identifying babies at risk requires integration of efforts by neonatology, ophthalmology, and nursing, a plan for setting up an effective program is presented by just such an interdisciplinary team (B Darlow, a neonatologist, C Gilbert, an ophthalmologist, and A Quiroga, a NICU nurse). They also emphasize the importance of collaboration with other health care professionals, funding organizations, administration, and policymakers.

One of the continuing challenges in ROP prevention is determining "ideal" protocols for oxygen treatment of premature babies. This thorny issue is addressed by Stenson and Fleck, who document our current state of knowledge and point out the continued research needed for the most commonly used drug in the NICU.

Several articles in this issue address the difficulty of balancing the number of ophthalmologists with expertise in detection and treatment of serious ROP and the fact that only a small percentage of babies at risk actually need treatment. There are exciting possibilities that are well along in development and may develop into clinically useful tools. Binenbaum reports here on the efforts to develop early indicators for ROP

Clin Perinatol 40 (2013) xvii–xviii
http://dx.doi.org/10.1016/j.clp.2013.04.001
0095-5108/13/$ – see front matter © 2013 Published by Elsevier Inc.

perinatology.theclinics.com

risk based on weight gain over the first weeks after birth. Wilson, Ells, and Fielder report important steps toward improving the utility of digital retinal imagining in at-risk babies. With quantitative analysis of the images, there is the potential for quick and reliable feedback to the baby's care team about the eye status of the baby and the timing for care and/or treatment.

Fortunately, there have been a number of strides toward understanding basic mechanisms of this iatrogenic disease. The work described by Smith, Hård, and Hellstromin in this edition of *Clinics in Perinatology* provides potential paths from the basic science laboratory to novel potential treatments for at-risk babies. The report by Maldonado and Toth outline the use of new technologies for understanding the complex ocular structure changes in the eyes of at-risk babies. Using this new knowledge opens the way for new potential methods of detection and even new treatments.

A perspective on the current "gold-standard" treatment for ROP is provided by Wallace and Wu, along with the complex question of the use of anti-VEGF drugs in premature babies.[3] This potential treatment should be the focus of intense scrutiny over the next decade with opinions strongly held both pro and con until a large clinical trail is undertaken with an adequate sample to define ocular and systemic treatment effects.

It is an exciting and challenging time in ROP as it becomes an increasingly global problem. This presents opportunities for international cooperation in the prevention of ROP blindness, but also highlights potential pitfalls when opportunities for improving care are not incorporated. New ways to detect and treat babies and eyes at risk are evolving rapidly and validation on these modalities is essential. Efforts must be made toward international collaboration and cooperation among all stakeholders in the prevention of ROP blindness.

Graham E. Quinn, MD, MSCE
Division of Ophthalmology
University of Pennsylvania Perelman School of Medicine
The Children's Hospital of Philadelphia
Wood Center, 1st Floor
Philadelphia, PA 19104, USA

Alistair R. Fielder, FRCP, FRCS, FRCOphth
Department of Optometry and Visual Science
City University
Northampton Square
London EC1V 0HB, United Kingdom

E-mail addresses:
QUINN@email.chop.edu (G.E. Quinn)
a.fielder@city.ac.uk (A.R. Fielder)

REFERENCES

1. Gilbert C, Fielder A, Gordillo L, et al. Characteristics of infants with severe retinopathy of prematurity in countries with low, moderate, and high levels of development: implications for screening programs. Pediatrics 2005;115:e518–25.
2. Gilbert C. Retinopathy of prematurity: a global perspective of the epidemics, population of babies at risk and implications for control. Early Hum Dev 2008;84: 77–82.
3. Mintz-Hittner HA, Kennedy KA, Chuang AZ. Efficacy of intravitreal bevacizumab for stage 3+ retinopathy of prematurity. New Engl J Med 2011;364:603–15.

Retinopathy of Prematurity-Incidence Today

Andrea Zin, MD, MSc, PhD[a],
Glen A. Gole, MD BS (NSW), FRANZCO, FRACS[b],*

KEYWORDS

- Retinopathy of prematurity • Retinopathy of prematurity incidence
- Childhood blindness • Retinopathy of prematurity detection

KEY POINTS

- Retinopathy of prematurity (ROP) is still a common cause of childhood blindness in high-income countries, although it no longer occurs in epidemic proportions.
- In middle-income countries, where there are often high rates of premature birth, ROP is now occurring in epidemic proportions (the third epidemic); it often occurs in babies of higher gestational age and birth weights than high-income countries, probably because of suboptimal neonatal care.
- If timely ROP detection and treatment programs are not put into place in middle-income countries, blindness from ROP is likely to increase because the survival of premature babies is increasing particularly in these countries.

INTRODUCTION: FIRST, SECOND, AND THIRD EPIDEMICS OF RETINOPATHY OF PREMATURITY

Retinopathy of prematurity (ROP) is a vasoproliferative retinopathy that affects the developing retinal vessels of premature infants. Despite being a treatable disorder, in its more severe forms, it can lead to traction retinal detachment and blindness. Because it is a disease of prematurity, it basically only occurs in those countries whose economy is developed or is developing to the stage whereby resuscitation of such infants is undertaken and neonatal care is in place.

ROP occurs worldwide except in countries with such high infant mortality rates (IMRs) that premature babies do not survive (eg, Sub-Saharan Africa). Globally, there are at least 50 000 children blind from ROP, which remains an important cause of childhood blindness in high-income countries, such as the United States, and is also emerging as a major cause of childhood blindness in middle-income economies,

[a] Clinical Research Unit, Fernandes Figueira Institute, Av Rui Barbosa 716, Flamengo, Rio de Janeiro 22250-020, Brazil; [b] Discipline of Paediatrics and Child Health, The University of Queensland, The Royal Children's Hospital, Brisbane, Queensland 4029, Australia
* Corresponding author.
E-mail address: g.gole@uq.edu.au

Clin Perinatol 40 (2013) 185–200
http://dx.doi.org/10.1016/j.clp.2013.02.001
0095-5108/13/$ – see front matter © 2013 Elsevier Inc. All rights reserved.
perinatology.theclinics.com

such as Latin America, Eastern Europe, India, and China.[1,2] The first epidemic of the disease occurred in the 1940s and 1950s with the advent of unmonitored oxygen therapy for the treatment of respiratory impairment in premature infants. At that time, ROP became the single most common cause of childhood blindness in high-income countries.[3] The unmonitored use of oxygen as a treatment of respiratory distress came to a close following a randomized controlled trial, which compared high and low oxygen treatment of premature infants.[4] This trial showed increased ROP in the high oxygen group. As a consequence, the use of oxygen was dramatically restricted, which led to a decrease in blindness owing to ROP; but this also caused an increase in mortality and morbidity (eg, cerebral palsy) over the succeeding 2 decades.[5] With the advent of neonatal intensive care units (NICUs) in the early 1970s, a second epidemic in high-income countries developed, which was controlled following improvements in neonatal intensive care and the introduction of retinal ablative therapy, first by means of cryotherapy[6,7] and thereafter by laser.[8] With rising standards of living and medical care in middle-income countries, particularly in the last 2 decades, improvement in the survival rate of premature infants followed. As a consequence, a third epidemic of ROP in these countries has ensued. This review compares the incidence of ROP across countries that present different levels of economic development and, indirectly, neonatal care.

ROP INCIDENCE WORLDWIDE

Most studies report ROP incidences[8–14] that are about 60% for babies less than 1500 g in nurseries in high-income countries. In middle-income countries, this figure is very variable depending on the birth and survival rates of premature infants and the fact that ROP occurs in much older and bigger babies than in high-income countries because of varying standards of neonatal care. Consequently, the authors do not consider the overall incidence of (any) ROP detected in nurseries as a useful yardstick in terms of the prevention of blindness measures because mild ROP, which is relatively common and is captured in incidence figures, almost always regresses without visual sequelae (ie, it is not sight threatening). However, severe ROP[12,14–47] (**Tables 1** and **2**), with the potential of blindness and the proven benefits of treatment, is a much more useful measure in terms of public health to estimate the magnitude of ROP in a particular population and helps to inform the setting of screening criteria. However, the direct comparison of rates can be difficult because different definitions of severe and treatable disease as well as different screening and study criteria are used. For example, many articles describe *severe ROP* as stages 3 to 5 which groups together stage 3,[48] which is a stage of active ROP (for which, in most countries with good ophthalmic care, treatment will be given), with stages 4 and 5, which are often end points of the disease process whether or not treatment has been undertaken. Nonetheless, the term *severe ROP* generally refers to a stage of the disease whereby sight is threatened and treatment may be offered, so the authors consider this to be a useful, if imprecise, term. As examples, the 2 largest therapeutic trials to date, The Multicenter Study of Cryotherapy of ROP (CRYO-ROP)[7] and the Early Treatment of Retinopathy of Prematurity trial (ETROP),[8] used slightly different definitions of ROP requiring treatment as did the Bevacizumab Eliminates the Angiogenic Threat of ROP (BEAT-ROP) study (**Box 1**).[49] The CRYO-ROP study, which involved more than 4000 preterm infants with birth weights (BWs) less than 1251 g, reported ROP of any stage in 65.8%. The incidence was higher in infants with BWs less than 750 g (90%) than in those weighing between 751 and 1000 g (78%) or 1001 to 1250 g (47%).[9] A decade after the CRYO-ROP study, the ETROP study disclosed a similar overall incidence

Table 1
Severe ROP incidence in high-income countries

Country	Study	Period	BW and/or GA Study Population	Number of NICUs	Number of Babies	Definition of Severe ROP	Severe ROP Incidence (%)
Australia	Gunn et al[14]	1992–2009	GA 23.0–25.6 wk	1	373	Stage 3 or more	15.0
Australia & New Zealand	Darlow et al,[15] ANZNN	1998–1999	GA <29 wk	29	2105	Stage 3 or more	9.4
Australia	Ahmed et al[10]	1998–2002	BW >1250 g GA 31–33 wk		906	Treatable ROP (CRYO-ROP)	0.0
Austria	Weber et al[16]	1999–2001	GA 22–26 wk	16	316	Stage 3 or more	16.0
Belgium	Allegaert,[17] The EpiBel Study	1999–2000	GA 22–26 wk	All units in Belgium	175	Stage 3 or more Treatable ROP (CRYO-ROP)	25.5 19.8
Canada	Shah et al,[18] Canadian Neonatal Network	1996–1997 (P1) 2006–2007 (P2)	GA <29 wk	15	1897 (P1) 1866 (P2)	Stage 2 or more	5.7 (P1) 3.9 (P2)
Croatia	Prpic et al[19]	1998–2002 (P1) 2003–2007 (P2)	BW <1500 g and GA ≤32 wk		226	Stage 3	30.6 (P1) 14.0 (P2)
Germany	Schwarz et al[20]	1978–1992 (P1) 1993–2007 (P2)	BW <1000 g	1	1473	Treatable ROP (CRYO-ROP, ETROP)	19.5 (P1) 14.8 (P2)
Kuwait	Wani et al[21]	Jan 2001–Aug 2003	BW <1501 g or GA ≤34 wk	1	599	Treatable ROP (stage 3, zone I or II, with 3 contiguous or 5 cumulative clock h of extraretinal proliferation and plus)	7.8

(continued on next page)

Table 1
(continued)

Country	Study	Period	BW and/or GA Study Population	Number of NICUs	Number of Babies	Definition of Severe ROP	Severe ROP Incidence (%)
Norway	Markestad et al,[22] on behalf of the Norwegian Extreme Prematurity Study Group	1999–2000	BW <1000 g	15	376	Treatable ROP (CRYO-ROP)	3.7
Saudi Arabia	Binkhathlan et al[23]	Jul 2003–Jul 2004	BW <2000 g and/or GA <36 wk	1	166	Treatable ROP (CRYO-ROP)	1.2
Saudi Arabia	Amer et al[24]	2009–2011	BW ≤1500 g and/or GA ≤32 wk	2	386	Treatable ROP	6.4
Singapore	Shah et al[25]	1988–2001	BW ≤1500 g	8	564	Stage 3 or more	8.0
Sweden	Austeng et al[11]	Apr 2009–Mar 2007	GA <27 wk	All units in Sweden	506	Stage 3–5 Treatable ROP (ETROP)	34.8 / 19.6
United Kingdom	Brennan et al[26]	Aug 1987–Oct 1998	1987–1990 BW ≤1500 g (P1) 1990–1999 BW ≤1500 g and/or GA <32 wk (P2)	Units in the Newcastle upon Tyne hospitals and in Gaeshead (North England)	484	Treatable ROP (CRYO-ROP)	5.2

Country	Study	Period	Criteria	No.	Network	N	Outcome	Prethreshold / Threshold
United States	Palmer et al,[9] CRYO-ROP Cooperative Group	Jan 1986–Nov 1987	BW <1251 g	23		4099		Prethreshold 6.0 Threshold 18.0
United States	Good et al,[8] ETROP Cooperative Group	Oct 2000–Sept 2002	BW <1251 g	26		6998	Treatable ROP (ETROP)	12.2
United States	Stoll et al,[27] Eunice Kennedy Shriver National Institute of Child Health and Human Development Neonatal Research Network	2003–2007	BW 401–1500 g and GA 22–28 wk	20		6866	Stage 3 or more Treatable ROP	16.0 12.0
United States	Mintz-Hittner et al,[49] BEAT-ROP Cooperative Group	Mar 2008–Aug 2010	BW <1500 g or GA <30 wk	15		?	Stage 3+ in zone I or II	
United States	Horbar et al,[28] Vermont-Oxford Neonatal Network	2009	BW 501–1500 g		Vermont-Oxford Neonatal Network	38 017	Stage 3–5	6.8

Abbreviations: ANZNN, Australian and New Zealand Neonatal Network; BEAT-ROP, Bevacizumab Eliminates the Angiogenic Threat of ROP; BW, birth weight; CRYO-ROP, Multicenter Study of Cryotherapy of ROP; ETROP, Early Treatment of Retinopathy of Prematurity; GA, gestational age; P1, period 1; P2, period 2.
Data from World Bank 2012. Available at: http://data.worldbank.org/about/country-classifications/country-and-lending-groups. Accessed March 23, 2013.

Table 2
Severe ROP incidence in middle- and low-income countries

Country	Study	Period	BW and/or GA Study Population	Number of NICUs	Number of Babies	Definition of Severe ROP	Severe ROP Incidence (%)
World Bank Country Groups by Income							
Upper middle income							
Argentina	Tavosnanska,[29] 2012 Neonatal Network of Public Hospitals of the City of Buenos Aires	2008–2010	BW 500–1499 g	15	1169	Treatable ROP	13.4
Brazil	Fortes Filho et al,[30] 2009	Oct 2002–Dec 2006	BW ≤1500 g and/or GA ≤32 wk	1	353	Treatable ROP (CRYO-ROP)	5.9
Brazil	Zin et al,[31] 2010	Jan 2004–Oct 2006	BW ≤2000 g and/or GA <37 wk	7	3437	Treatable ROP (ETROP)	3.4
China	Li et al,[32] 2012	2009–2010	BW ≤2000 g or GA ≤34 wk	1	2185	Any stage ROP 3	13.1 1.3
Colombia	Zuluaga et al,[33] 2006	Jan 2001–Dec 2005	BW <1500 g and < GA ≤32 wk	1	1138	Treatable ROP (CRYO-ROP)	8.0
Iran	Saeidi et al,[34] 2009	April 2005–March 2006	BW ≤1500 g or GA ≤32 wk	1	45	ROP any stage	8.5
Lithuania	Jakuskiene et al,[35] 2011	2003–2005	BW ≤1500 g and GA ≤32 wk	1	338	Treatable ROP	4.2
Romania	Vatavu et al,[36] 2010	Sept 2002–Dec 2007	BW ≤2000 g and/or GA ≤34 wk	1	1783	Treatable ROP	15.2
Serbia	Knezevic et al,[37] 2011	Jun 2006–Dec 2009	BW <2000 g or GA <37 wk	1	478	Treatable ROP	21.3

South Africa	Delport et al,[38] 2002	Feb 1999–Dec 1999	BW ≤1500 g	1	94	Treatable ROP (CRYO-ROP)	4.3
Turkey	Akkoyun et al,[39] 2006	May 2002–Jun 2004	GA <34 wk	1	88	Stage 3	29.5
Lower middle income							
India	Charan et al,[12] 1995	1993	BW ≤1700 g	1	165	Stage 3 or more	12.8
India	Gopal et al,[40] 1995	Nov 1992–Jan 1994	BW ≤2000 g	1	50	Treatable ROP (CRYO-ROP)	16.0
India	Vinekar et al,[42] 2007	Jun 1993–May 2003	BW >1250 g	1	138	Treatable ROP (CRYO-ROP) + stages 4 and 5	44.9
India	Varughese et al,[41] 2001	Jun 1999–May 2000	BW <1500 g and GA <34 wk	1	79	Treatable ROP (CRYO-ROP)	6.3
India	Jalali et al,[43] 2006	Oct 1999–Dec 2002	BW <2000 g GA <36 wk	2	1083	Threshold ROP, prethreshold ROP zone 1 stage 4A or more	11.0
India	Hungi et al,[44] 2012	Dec 2008–May 2010	BW ≤2000 g and/or GA ≤34 wk	1	118	Treatable ROP (ETROP)	10.2
Pakistan	Taqui et al,[45] 2008	March 2003–Sept 2006	BW ≤1500 g and/or GA ≤32 wk	1	68	Treatable ROP (CRYO-ROP)	20.6
Vietnam	Phan et al,[46] 2003	2001	BW ≤1500 g and/or GA ≤33 wk	1	225	Treatable ROP (CRYO-ROP)	9.3
Low income							
Bangladesh	Ahmed et al,[47] 2008	Dec 1998–July 2003	GA <33 wk	1	114	ROP any stage	4.4

Abbreviations: BW, birth weight; CRYO-ROP, Multicenter Study of Cryotherapy of ROP; ETROP, Early Treatment of Retinopathy of Prematurity; GA, gestational age; P1, period 1; P2, period 2.

Data from World Bank 2012. Available at: http://data.worldbank.org/about/country-classifications/country-and-lending-groups.

Box 1
Criteria for severe ROP (ie, treatment recommended)

CRYO-ROP Study[6,7]

- Five or more contiguous or 8 cumulative 30° sectors (clock hours) of stage
- 3+ retinopathy of prematurity in zone 1 or 2

ETROP Study[8]

- Type 1 ROP
  - Zone I, any stage ROP with plus disease
  - Zone 1, stage 3 ROP without plus disease
  - Zone II, stage 2 or 3 with plus disease

BEAT-ROP Study[49]

- Stage 3+ ROP in zone I or posterior zone II

(68%).[8] A recent multicenter report from North America of newborns with a gestational age (GA) of 22 to 28 weeks and BWs of 401 to 1500 g gives an overall ROP (any stage) incidence of 59% with a 16% incidence of severe ROP.[27] Beginning with the CRYO-ROP study, many articles have reported that the incidence of ROP increases as the BW and GA decrease.[14,15,25,30,39]

Considered globally, the BWs and GAs of babies at risk varies from high- to middle- and low-income countries, with many babies from middle-income countries with BWs more than 1500 g and GAs greater than 32 weeks developing disease that requires treatment.[50] In middle-income countries, children who develop blinding ROP in different units, even in the same city, may have distinctly different BWs and GAs,[31] indicating that improvements in neonatal care are not uniformly distributed. The picture in developing economies seems to be related to the quality of neonatal care available. Some examples that display this are India, some Eastern European countries, and Latin America.

India

In India, large, relatively mature babies with BWs more than 1500 g and GAs more than 34 weeks or so have been reported to have high incidences of severe ROP since the early 1990s. For example, Charan and colleagues[12] reported in 1995 an overall incidence of 47% ROP in their babies with BWs of 1700 g or less, with an incidence of 12.8% requiring treatment; this figure has changed little over the 15 years or so.[40,43,44] In a retrospective study of 138 patients with BWs more than 1250 gm referred for ROP examination, Vinekar and colleagues[42] reported that 45% had threshold or worse ROP, demonstrating that severe ROP occurs in bigger babies in India.

In a telephone survey of Indian pediatricians, referral rates for ROP screening were reported to be very low, with 34% not referring at all.[51] The most common reason was the nonavailability of trained ophthalmologists. Lack of screening was a causative factor for stage 5 ROP in nearly 90% of affected babies reported by one referral center.[52]

Supplemental unblended oxygen was considered a factor in causing aggressive posterior ROP (AP-ROP)[48] in a case series of larger Indian babies.[53] Fluorescein angiography in these children showed massive capillary dropout suggestive of the vaso-obliteration seen in animal models of ROP whereby the experimental disease is produced by oxygen overdose.[54] Severe ROP occurring in some Indian babies has been reported to have a combination of features of both a neovascular ridge and flat neovascular tissue in the posterior pole (hybrid ROP),[55] which is hard to classify in terms of the disease described in high-income economies.[48]

The authors speculate that the number of infants potentially blind from ROP in India alone will accumulate, over a few years, to approach the 50 000 ROP blind worldwide figure previously estimated[1] unless widespread screening and treatment are introduced (ignoring improvements in neonatal care). The authors base this on the following assumptions: the 2012 birth rate in India of 27.2 million per year (United Nations' [UN] estimate); a 13% prematurity rate,[56] with perhaps half of these children at risk (6.5%); 40% of premature infants having access to care, with a 75% survival overall (Clare Gilbert, personal communication, 2013); a 10% incidence of severe ROP; a 50% unfavorable outcome in an untreated group[7] (CRYO-ROP control group); and a 15% failure rate with laser treatment (poor visual outcomes from the ETROP study). The authors have no basis to speculate about the impact of anti–vascular endothelial growth factor treatment of ROP[49] in this context.

The calculation is as follows: $27\,200\,000 \times 6.5\% \times 40.0\% \times 75.0\% \times 10.0\% = 53\,040$ infants with severe ROP per year; without treatment, $53\,040 \times 50\% = 25\,520$ infants blind from ROP; with laser treatment, $53\,040 \times 15\% = 7956$ infants blind from ROP.

The difference between offering and not offering ROP screening and laser treatment is 17 564 blind infants each year in India alone.

Eastern Europe

In the former Soviet Bloc countries, the incidence of severe ROP varies from more prosperous countries where figures are similar to Western countries (eg, Lithuania[35]) to other countries (Croatia, Romania, Serbia) where the rates are much higher and affect babies with higher BWs and GAs, which is more typical of middle-income countries.[19,36,37]

Latin America

Although Latin American countries are middle-income economies, the region, together with Sub-Saharan Africa, is one of the most unequal in the world.[57] The varying levels of socioeconomic development impact on the health care infrastructure, availability, and patient access to care. This scenario will reflect on the causes of childhood blindness across the region. Overall, ROP has been reported as an important cause of childhood blindness in several Latin American countries, with the proportion of children blind from ROP varying from 4.1% in Guatemala to 38.6% in Cuba.[58]

In Mexico, in a survey performed during a national neonatology congress in 2007, 60% of responders reported that a ROP detection and treatment program was not available in their units. Barriers identified for its implementation were lack of skilled ophthalmologists, access to technology and equipment, economic resources, and institutional support for the time devoted to ROP care.[59] A blind school survey performed in 2 institutions in Guadalajara, in 2009, found that ROP was the main cause of childhood blindness (34.7%), and only 53% of NICUs in the city had implemented a regular ROP examination and treatment program.[60]

The picture was very similar in Cali, Colombia, where ROP was also the main cause of childhood blindness (33.8%). Once again, there was no ROP program implemented in the city.[61]

The BW and GA of babies presenting severe and treatable disease also have a wide variation, which may reflect the diverse quality of neonatal care provided. In a 7-year single-unit study in Mexico, 5% of babies with treatable disease showed BWs of 1501 to 2000 g.[13] In Argentina, 27% of treated cases from 27 NICUs had BWs more than 1500 g. The same investigators stated that only 1 out of 900 live births was treated; however, this figure could be an underestimate because not all premature babies had access to diagnosis.[31,62–65]

Reported rates of treatable ROP varied from 19.1% in Lima, Peru,[63] to 5.9% in a unit in the South of Brazil.[66]

Several studies indicate the need for wider screening criteria in middle-income economies as large, more mature infants are developing treatable ROP. Gilbert and colleagues[50] showed that, overall, 13% of infants from several middle- and low-income countries would not have been examined if UK screening criteria had been adopted. In Beijing, China, Chen and Li[67] showed that 16.2% of infants who developed severe ROP (ie, disease needing laser treatment or surgery for stage 4 or 5 ROP) exceeded the UK screening criteria and 30.4% exceeded the US screening criteria.[67] In India, Jalali and colleagues[43] reported that 8% exceeded the UK criteria and 13% exceeded the US criteria. Two studies from Brazil also stated the need for wider screening criteria because a considerable percentage of infants examined who developed treatable disease would not have been examined if UK screening criteria had been used.[31,68]

Regional incidence of ROP and its relationship to IMRs and rates of premature birth
The incidence of blindness from ROP varies enormously from country to country.[1] Gilbert reported that it seems that the risk of ROP-related blindness is correlated with IMRs,[1] which, themselves, reflect the level of access to and the quality of health care and the level of socioeconomic development. Countries with IMRs greater than 60 per 1000 live births, generally low and lower middle-income economies, usually do not have neonatal intensive care facilities and often lack even basic facilities for pregnant women, so preterm babies do not survive. For example, a childhood blindness survey in Yemen reported no cases of ROP.[69] Those countries with IMRs less than 9 per 1000 live births are high-income economies that count on strong health systems that allow access of premature babies to good quality neonatal care, including diagnosis and treatment of severe ROP. Countries with IMRs of 9 to 60 per 1000 live births now represent the highest risk of ROP blindness because many babies at risk survive in neonatal nurseries where oxygen use may be poorly monitored, ROP diagnostic and treatment programs are not consistently in place,[1] and even screening protocols are not widely followed.[51,70] Those countries are usually middle-income economies. ROP is now considered the most common cause of blindness in Latin American countries,[71] although cerebral vision impairment is much more prevalent as a cause of childhood blindness in developed countries, such as the United States[2] and the United Kingdom,[72] especially in survivors of prematurity. Refractive errors and strabismus are also more common in premature infants.[73]

IMRs have decreased substantially since 1990. In the developing countries, the IMR declined from 97 deaths per 1000 live births in 1990 to 63 in 2010, representing a decline of 35%. Worldwide, even with the population growth, the number of deaths in children less than 5 years old decreased from more than 12 million in 1990 to 7.6 million in 2010.[74] This decrease in IMRs might represent an increased risk of blindness from ROP in survivors who are also premature.

RATES OF PREMATURE BIRTH, MILLENNIUM DEVELOPMENT GOALS, AND ROP

An emerging issue with the third epidemic of ROP is that rates of premature birth are rising in almost all countries when reliable data are collected. Globally, more than 10% of babies are born preterm (GA <37 weeks), which translates into more than 15 million premature babies annually worldwide.[56] Most infants (84%) are moderately premature (32–37 weeks); in middle-income economies, they are at high risk of developing blinding ROP. A further 10.4% of premature infants are born between 28 and 32 weeks and 5.2% are born at less than 28 weeks.[56] In low-income countries, babies born at 28 to 32 weeks still have a 50% mortality because of a lack of lack of warmth, basic support for breastfeeding, and facilities to treat immediate respiratory difficulties and infection.[74]

Almost all of the countries with rates of premature birth of more than 15% also have high IMRs. Ten countries account for 60% of all preterm births. These countries are (in order) India, China, Nigeria, Pakistan, Indonesia, United States, Bangladesh, Philippines, Congo, and Brazil.[74]

The presence of the United States on this list may reflect economic differences between racial groups as well as regional differences regarding access to neonatal care. In middle-income countries, ROP is now an important cause of childhood blindness[60,75] and still remains a common cause of childhood blindness even in high-income countries.[2]

The decrease of IMR is the fourth goal of the Millennium Development Goals (MDGs), the UN's action plan to raise the world's population out of extreme poverty, and its consequences, by 2015. Worldwide, governments of low- and middle-income countries are engaged to achieve the MDGs.[76] The wide implementation of NICUs combined with the advances in neonatal care over the past decades, such as antenatal steroid and surfactant therapy, protective ventilatory care, and nutrition strategies, have contributed to an important improvement in the survival of very low birth weight infants in several developed and developing economies (eg, United States[28] and Brazil).[77] However, in some middle-income countries, the improvements in maternal health and newborn survival overall are being affected by an increase in premature births, caused in part by inaccurate ultrasound scans, and the increase of labor induction and caesarean sections for nonmedical reasons.[78] These nonmedical reasons for inducing delivery particularly cause an increase in birth rates of moderately premature infants (32–37 weeks' GA),[56] which is the high-risk group for ROP in middle-income countries. Simple, often low-cost measures, including reducing nonmedical reasons for delivery, are predicted to reduce the rate of premature births if adopted widely.[79]

The improved survival in those middle-income economies has increased the population at risk of developing treatable ROP, which may represent a challenge in those countries where timely ROP screening and treatment are not in place. In high-income countries, there seems to have been a continuous decrease of the prevalence of blinding ROP over the last decade or so coincident with improved survival.[28] This decrease may be caused by a combination of incremental improvements in neonatal care, widespread screening for ROP, and the timing of laser treatment before irreversible retinal scarring occurs. However, these improvements in neonatal outcomes in high-income countries have not been uniform.[18,20,27]

Improved quality of neonatal care not only impacts on survival but also morbidity rates.[15,31] In middle-income economies, although survival is improving constantly, morbidity rates are still higher than in high-income countries, demonstrating that that those countries need to improve their quality of neonatal care even more.

SUMMARY

ROP in high-income countries now occurs, mostly in extreme low birth weight infants. In those countries, the incidence of ROP seems to have declined incrementally over the last few decades. But in middle-income-countries, high rates of premature birth and increasing resuscitation of premature infants, often with suboptimal standards of care, have resulted in a third epidemic of ROP. Improved maternal and neonatal care, ROP screening guidelines appropriate to middle-income countries, and widespread timely treatment are urgently called for to control this third epidemic.

ACKNOWLEDGMENTS

G.G. would like to acknowledge Prof Rajvardhan Azad from the Dr RP Center at the All India Institute of Medical Sciences, New Delhi, India for the inspiration about the potential numbers of Indian babies blinded by ROP and Professor Clare Gilbert from the London School of Hygiene and Tropical Medicine, London, UK for her generous assistance and comments on the calculations (for which G.G. takes full responsibility).

REFERENCES

1. Gilbert C. Retinopathy of prematurity: a global perspective of the epidemics, population of babies at risk and implications for control. Early Hum Dev 2008; 84(2):77–82.
2. Kong L, Fry M, Al-Samarraie M, et al. An update on progress and the changing epidemiology of causes of childhood blindness worldwide. J AAPOS 2012;16(6): 501–7.
3. Silverman WA. Retrolental fibroplasia: a modern parable. New York: Grune and Stratton, Inc; 1980. p. 207.
4. Kinsey VE, Hemphill FM. Etiology of retrolental fibroplasia and preliminary report of the Cooperative Study of Retrolental Fibroplasia. Trans Am Acad Ophthalmol Otolaryngol 1955;59:15–24.
5. Bolton DP, Cross KW. Further observations on cost of preventing retrolental fibroplasia. Lancet 1974;1(7855):445–8.
6. Group CfRoPC. Multicenter trial of cryotherapy for retinopathy of prematurity. Three-month outcome. Cryotherapy for Retinopathy of Prematurity Cooperative Group. Arch Ophthalmol 1990;108(2):195–204.
7. CfRoPC Group. Multicenter trial of cryotherapy for retinopathy of prematurity. One-year outcome–structure and function. Cryotherapy for Retinopathy of Prematurity Cooperative Group. Arch Ophthalmol 1990;108(10):1408–16.
8. Good WV, Hardy RJ, Dobson V, et al. The incidence and course of retinopathy of prematurity: findings from the early treatment for retinopathy of prematurity study. Pediatrics 2005;116(1):15–23.
9. Palmer EA, Flynn JT, Hardy RJ, et al. Incidence and early course of retinopathy of prematurity. The Cryotherapy for Retinopathy of Prematurity Cooperative Group. Ophthalmology 1991;98(11):1628–40.
10. Ahmed MA, Duncan M, Kent A, et al. Incidence of retinopathy of prematurity requiring treatment in infants born greater than 30 weeks' gestation and with a birthweight greater than 1250 g from 1998 to 2002: a regional study. J Paediatr Child Health 2006;42(6):337–40.
11. Austeng D, Kallen KB, Ewald UW, et al. Incidence of retinopathy of prematurity in infants born before 27 weeks' gestation in Sweden. Arch Ophthalmol 2009; 127(10):1315–9.
12. Charan R, Dogra MR, Gupta A, et al. The incidence of retinopathy of prematurity in a neonatal care unit. Indian J Ophthalmol 1995;43(3):123–6.

13. Flores-Santos R, Hernandez-Cabrera MA, Henandez-Herrera RJ, et al. Screening for retinopathy of prematurity: results of a 7-year study of underweight newborns. Arch Med Res 2007;38(4):440–3.
14. Gunn DJ, Cartwright DW, Gole GA. Incidence of retinopathy of prematurity in extremely premature infants over an 18-year period. Clin Experiment Ophthalmol 2012;40(1):93–9.
15. Darlow BA, Hutchinson JL, Henderson-Smart DJ, et al. Prenatal risk factors for severe retinopathy of prematurity among very preterm infants of the Australian and New Zealand Neonatal Network. Pediatrics 2005;115(4):990–6.
16. Weber C, Weninger M, Klebermass K, et al. Mortality and morbidity in extremely preterm infants (22 to 26 weeks of gestation): Austria 1999-2001. Wien Klin Wochenschr 2005;117(21–22):740–6.
17. Allegaert K. Threshold retinopathy at threshold of viability: the EpiBel study. Br J Ophthalmol 2004;88(2):239–42.
18. Shah PS, Sankaran K, Aziz K, et al. Outcomes of preterm infants <29 weeks gestation over 10-year period in Canada: a cause for concern? J Perinatol 2012;32(2):132–8.
19. Prpić I, Mahulja-Stamenković V, Kovacević D, et al. Prevalence of severe retinopathy of prematurity in a geographically defined population in Croatia. Coll Antropol 2011;35(Suppl 2):69–72.
20. Schwarz EC, Grauel EL, Wauer RR. Kein Anstieg von Inzidenz, Therapie- und Erblindungsrate der Retinopathia praematurorum in einem universitaren Perinatalzentrum Level 1-eine prospektive Beobachtungsstudie von 1978–2007. [No increase of incidence of retinopathy of prematurity and improvement of its outcome in a university perinatal centre level III - a prospective observational study from 1978 to 2007]. Klin Monbl Augenheilkd 2011;228(3):208–19 [in German].
21. Wani VB, Kumar N, Sabti K, et al. Results of screening for retinopathy of prematurity in a large nursery in Kuwait: incidence and risk factors. Indian J Ophthalmol 2010;58(3):204–8.
22. Markestad T, Kaaresen PI, Ronnestad A, et al. Early death, morbidity, and need of treatment among extremely premature infants. Pediatrics 2005;115(5):1289–98.
23. Binkhathlan AA, Almahmoud LA, Saleh MJ, et al. Retinopathy of prematurity in Saudi Arabia: incidence, risk factors, and the applicability of current screening criteria. Br J Ophthalmol 2008;92(2):167–9.
24. Amer M, Jafri WH, Nizami AM, et al. Retinopathy of prematurity: are we missing any infant with retinopathy of prematurity? Br J Ophthalmol 2012;96(8):1052–5.
25. Shah VA, Yeo CL, Ling YL, et al. Incidence, risk factors of retinopathy of prematurity among very low birth weight infants in Singapore. Ann Acad Med Singapore 2005;34(2):169–78.
26. Brennan R, Gnanaraj L, Cottrell DG. Retinopathy of prematurity in practice. I: screening for threshold disease. Eye (Lond) 2003;17(2):183–8.
27. Stoll BJ, Hansen NI, Bell EF, et al. Neonatal outcomes of extremely preterm infants from the NICHD Neonatal Research Network. Pediatrics 2010;126(3):443–56.
28. Horbar JD, Carpenter JH, Badger GJ, et al. Mortality and neonatal morbidity among infants 501 to 1500 grams from 2000 to 2009. Pediatrics 2012;129(6):1019–26.
29. Tavosnanska J. Morbimortalidad de recién nacidos con menos de 1500 gramos asistidos en hospitales públicos de la Ciudad de Buenos Aires. Arch Argent Pediatr 2012;110(5):394–403.

30. Fortes Filho JB, Eckert GU, Procianoy L, et al. Incidence and risk factors for retinopathy of prematurity in very low and in extremely low birth weight infants in a unit-based approach in southern Brazil. Eye (Lond) 2009;23(1):25–30.
31. Zin AA, Moreira ME, Bunce C, et al. Retinopathy of prematurity in 7 neonatal units in Rio de Janeiro: screening criteria and workload implications. Pediatrics 2010; 126(2):e410–7.
32. Li QP, Wang Z, Li YY, et al. Retinopathy of prematurity screening in 2185 premature infants. Zhonghua Yan Ke Za Zhi 2012;48(10):903–7 [in Chinese].
33. Zuluaga C, Llanos G, Torres J. Effects of the screening program on ROP in Cali, Colombia. Acta Med Lituan 2006;13(3):176–8.
34. Saeidi R, Hashemzadeh A, Ahmadi S, et al. Prevalence and predisposing factors of retinopathy of prematurity in very low-birth-weight infants discharged from NICU. Iran J Pediatr 2009;19(1):59–63.
35. Jakuskiene R, Vollmer B, Saferis V, et al. Neonatal outcomes of very preterm infants admitted to a tertiary center in Lithuania between the years 2003 and 2005. Eur J Pediatr 2011;170(10):1293–303.
36. Vătavu I, Nascutzy C, Ciomârtan T, et al. Retinopathy of prematurity–screening results. Oftalmologia 2010;54(1):110–7 [in Romanian].
37. Knezević S, Stojanović N, Oros A, et al. Analysis of risk factors in the development of retinopathy of prematurity. Srp Arh Celok Lek 2011;139(7–8):433–8 [in Serbian].
38. Delport SD, Swanepoel JC, Odendaal PJ, et al. Incidence of retinopathy of prematurity in very-low-birth-weight infants born at Kalafong Hospital, Pretoria. S Afr Med J 2002;92(12):986–90.
39. Akkoyun I, Oto S, Yilmaz G, et al. Risk factors in the development of mild and severe retinopathy of prematurity. J AAPOS 2006;10(5):449–53.
40. Gopal L, Sharma T, Ramachandran S, et al. Retinopathy of prematurity: a study. Indian J Ophthalmol 1995;43(2):59–61.
41. Varughese S, Jain S, Gupta N, et al. Magnitude of the problem of retinopathy of prematurity. Experience in a large maternity unit with a medium size level-3 nursery. Indian J Ophthalmol 2001;49(3):187–8.
42. Vinekar A, Dogra MR, Sangtam T, et al. Retinopathy of prematurity in Asian Indian babies weighing greater than 1250 grams at birth: ten year data from a tertiary care center in a developing country. Indian J Ophthalmol 2007;55(5):331–6.
43. Jalali S, Matalia J, Hussain A, et al. Modification of screening criteria for retinopathy of prematurity in India and other middle-income countries. Am J Ophthalmol 2006;141(5):966–8.
44. Hungi B, Vinekar A, Datti N, et al. Retinopathy of prematurity in a rural neonatal intensive care unit in South India–a prospective study. Indian J Pediatr 2012; 79(7):911–5.
45. Taqui AM, Syed R, Chaudhry TA, et al. Retinopathy of prematurity: frequency and risk factors in a tertiary care hospital in Karachi, Pakistan. J Pak Med Assoc 2008; 58(4):186–90.
46. Phan MH, Nguyen PN, Reynolds JD. Incidence and severity of retinopathy of prematurity in Vietnam, a developing middle-income country. J Pediatr Ophthalmol Strabismus 2003;40(4):208–12.
47. Ahmed AS, Muslima H, Anwar KS, et al. Retinopathy of prematurity in Bangladeshi neonates. J Trop Pediatr 2008;54(5):333–9.
48. International Committee for the Classification of Retinopathy of Prematurity. The international classification of retinopathy of prematurity revisited. Arch Ophthalmol 2005;123(7):991–9.

49. Mintz-Hittner HA, Kennedy KA, Chuang AZ, BEAT-ROP Cooperative Group. Efficacy of intravitreal bevacizumab for stage 3+ retinopathy of prematurity. N Engl J Med 2011;364(7):603–15.
50. Gilbert C, Fielder A, Gordillo L, et al. Characteristics of infants with severe retinopathy of prematurity in countries with low, moderate, and high levels of development: implications for screening programs. Pediatrics 2005;115(5):e518–25.
51. Patwardhan SD, Azad R, Gogia V, et al. Prevailing clinical practices regarding screening for retinopathy of prematurity among pediatricians in India: a pilot survey. Indian J Ophthalmol 2011;59(6):427–30.
52. Sanghi G, Dogra MR, Katoch D, et al. Demographic profile of infants with stage 5 retinopathy of prematurity in North India: implications for screening. Ophthalmic Epidemiol 2011;18(2):72–4.
53. Shah PK, Narendran V, Kalpana N. Aggressive posterior retinopathy of prematurity in large preterm babies in South India. Arch Dis Child Fetal Neonatal Ed 2012; 97(5):F371–5.
54. Stahl A, Connor KM, Sapieha P, et al. The mouse retina as an angiogenesis model. Invest Ophthalmol Vis Sci 2010;51(6):2813–26.
55. Sanghi G, Dogra MR, Dogra M, et al. A hybrid form of retinopathy of prematurity. Br J Ophthalmol 2012;96(4):519–22.
56. Blencowe H, Cousens S, Oestergaard MZ, et al. National, regional, and worldwide estimates of preterm birth rates in the year 2010 with time trends since 1990 for selected countries: a systematic analysis and implications. Lancet 2012;379(9832):2162–72.
57. Lopez JH, Perry G. Inequality in Latin America: determinants and consequences. Washington, DC: The World Bank; 2008.
58. Gilbert C, Rahi J, Eckstein M, et al. Retinopathy of prematurity in middle-income countries. Lancet 1997;350:12–4.
59. Zepeda Romero LC, Gutierrez Padilla JA, De la Fuente-Torres MA, et al. Detection and treatment for retinopathy of prematurity in Mexico: need for effective programs. J AAPOS 2008;12(3):225–6.
60. Zepeda-Romero LC, Barrera-de-Leon JC, Camacho-Choza C, et al. Retinopathy of prematurity as a major cause of severe visual impairment and blindness in children in schools for the blind in Guadalajara city, Mexico. Br J Ophthalmol 2011;95(11):1502–5.
61. Zuluaga C, Sierra MV, Asprilla E. Causas de ceguera infantil en Cali, Colombia. Colomb Med 2005;36:235.
62. Lomuto CC, Galina L, Brussa M, et al. Epidemiologia de la retinopatia del prematuro en servicios publicos de la Argentina durante 2008. [Epidemiology of retinopathy of prematurity in public services from Argentina during 2008]. Arch Argent Pediatr 2010;108(1):24–30 [in Spanish].
63. Turkowsky JD, Cervantes AC, Rocha PV, et al. Incidence of retinopathy of prematurity (ROP) and its evolution in the population preterms of very low birth weight survivors and that was discharged from the Instituto Especializado Materno Perinatal of Lima. Rev Peru Pediatr 2007;60(2):88–92 [in Spanish].
64. Restrepo MM, Guzman AH, Gomez JH, et al. Epidemiología de la retinopatía del prematuroen Medellín, 2003-2008. Iatreia 2011;24(3):25–258 [in Spanish].
65. Fernández YG, Ragi RM, Rivero MR, et al. Incidencia de la retinopatía de la prematuridad. Rev Cubana Pediatr 2007;79(2):1–6 [in Spanish].
66. Fortes Filho JB, Eckert GU, Valiatti FB, et al. Prevalence of retinopathy of prematurity: an institutional cross-sectional study of preterm infants in Brazil. Rev Panam Salud Publica 2009;26(3):216–20.

67. Chen Y, Li X. Characteristics of severe retinopathy of prematurity patients in China: a repeat of the first epidemic? Br J Ophthalmol 2006;90(3):268–71.
68. Filho JB, Barros CK, da Costa MC, et al. Results of a program for the prevention of blindness caused by retinopathy of prematurity in southern Brazil. J Pediatr (Rio J) 2007;83(3):209–16.
69. Bamashmus MA, Al-Akily SA. Profile of childhood blindness and low vision in Yemen: a hospital-based study. East Mediterr Health J 2010;16(4):425–8.
70. Available at: http://HDR_2011_EN_Table3.pdf. Accessed March 23, 2013.
71. Furtado JM, Lansingh VC, Carter MJ, et al. Causes of blindness and visual impairment in Latin America. Surv Ophthalmol 2012;57(2):149–77.
72. Crofts BJ, King R, Johnson A. The contribution of low birth weight to severe vision loss in a geographically defined population. Br J Ophthalmol 1998;82(1):9–13.
73. O'Connor AR, Wilson CM, Fielder AR. Ophthalmological problems associated with preterm birth. Eye (Lond) 2007;21(10):1254–60.
74. Howson CP, Kinney MV, Lawn JE, editors. March of Dimes P, Save the Children, WHO. Born too soon: the global action report on preterm birth. Geneva (Switzerland): World Health Organisation; 2012.
75. Dandona R, Dandona L. Childhood blindness in India: a population based perspective. Br J Ophthalmol 2003;87(3):263–5.
76. Nations U. The Millennium Development Goals report 2012. New York: United Nations; 2012.
77. Victora CG, Aquino EM, do Carmo Leal M, et al. Maternal and child health in Brazil: progress and challenges. Lancet 2011;377(9780):1863–76.
78. Barros FC, Victora CG, Barros AJ, et al. The challenge of reducing neonatal mortality in middle-income countries: findings from three Brazilian birth cohorts in 1982, 1993, and 2004. Lancet 2005;365(9462):847–54.
79. Chang HH, Larson J, Blencowe H, et al. Preventing preterm births: analysis of trends and potential reductions with interventions in 39 countries with very high human development index. Lancet 2013;381:223–34.

The Biology of Retinopathy of Prematurity
How Knowledge of Pathogenesis Guides Treatment

Lois E. Smith, MD, PhD[a],*, Anna-Lena Hard, MD, PhD[b],
Ann Hellström, MD, PhD[b],*

KEYWORDS

- Oxygen • IGF-1 • Omega-3 polyunsaturated fatty acids • Postnatal weight gain
- Erythropoietin

KEY POINTS

- Review the molecular pathogenesis of retinopathy of prematurity (ROP).
- Understand the role of the hypoxia-induced growth factors, particularly vascular endothelial growth factor, in the normal development of the retinal vasculature.
- Understand the contribution of factors lacking after preterm birth, nutrition, insulinlike growth factor 1 and polyunsaturated fatty acids, in normal retinal development.
- Describe clinical applications for the prevention/treatment of ROP, which have emerged from molecular studies.
- Appreciate the importance of neonatal weight gain as a predictor for the development of ROP.

INTRODUCTION

Retinopathy of prematurity (ROP) occurs because the retina of a preterm infant at birth is incompletely vascularized, and if the postnatal environment does not match the in utero environment that supported retinal development, the vessels and neural retina will not grow normally. Risk factors determined from many clinical studies and animal studies fall into 2 categories[1]:

L.E. Smith, A. Hellström: These authors contributed equally to the work.
[a] Department of Ophthalmology, Children's Hospital Boston, Harvard Medical School, Fegan 4, 300 Longwood Avenue, Boston, MA 02115, USA; [b] Section of Pediatric Ophthalmology, The Queen Silvia Children's Hospital, The Sahlgrenska Academy at University of Gothenburg, Göteborg S-416 85, Sweden
* Corresponding authors.
E-mail addresses: Lois.Smith@childrens.harvard.edu; ann.hellstrom@medfak.gu.se

Clin Perinatol 40 (2013) 201–214
http://dx.doi.org/10.1016/j.clp.2013.02.002
0095-5108/13/$ – see front matter © 2013 Elsevier Inc. All rights reserved.
perinatology.theclinics.com

1. Prenatal factors
   Those that reflect the degree of incomplete neurovascular development at birth indicating the susceptibility of the retina to harm
   a. Gestational age at birth
   b. Birth weight
2. Postnatal factors
   Factors after preterm birth that differ from the in utero environment of the third trimester and therefore do not match the extrauterine needs of the baby and prevent resumption of normal retinal neurovascular growth after birth:
   a. Exposure to oxygen, which is higher and/or more variable than that found during gestation that alters the oxygen-regulated growth factors
   b. Loss of the maternal-fetal interaction resulting in
      Increased metabolic demands[2] in the face of loss of nutrition (including essential fatty acids)
      Decreased IGF-I levels and loss of other factors resulting in poor postnatal growth and weight gain.[3–5]

Much of the authors' understanding of ROP has come from observations in the clinic, followed by animal studies to determine pathogenesis, which then are played out in clinical intervention studies resulting in changes in clinical practice. Optimally this cycle continues to refine patient care.

ROP was first described as "retrolental fibroplasia" by Terry in 1942.[6] In 1952, Patz and colleagues demonstrated in a clinical study the association between oxygen and ROP.[7] In an experimental kitten model,[8] Ashton then established the concepts of oxygen toxicity and vessel loss (phase I) followed by hypoxia-mediated vasoproliferation (phase II). Thus these studies characterized ROP as a 2-phased disease of preterm infants with initial cessation of vessel growth caused by exposure to high levels of oxygen and loss of formed vessels followed by pathologic neovascularization of the retina. As a result of these findings, oxygen use was severely curtailed for a time, and although ROP incidence decreased, many infants died as a result.[9]

The balance between sufficient supplemental oxygen to prevent death versus minimal oxygen to prevent ROP has still not been settled for premature infants at different gestational (GA) and postmenstrual ages (PMAs) despite a large number of clinical studies addressing aspects of the question.[10] The effect of supplemental oxygen use in phase I and phase II of ROP in these studies suggests that high oxygen saturation levels in phase I are a significant risk factor, and oxygen supplementation in phase II may reduce ROP risk slightly but may also increase lung disease.[11,12] These studies although hinting at the best use are not yet definitive, and we await a clinical study that will better inform optimal use of oxygen at different GA, different PMA.

ROP persists as a major cause of blindness in children despite better oxygen monitoring[13,14] because neonatal practices improve and infants at earlier GAs survive, with extreme retinal immaturity at birth.[15] The immature retina is susceptible not only to oxygen levels higher than those in utero but also to variable oxygen tensions and to lack of growth factors and nutrients normally provided in utero, all of which cause vessel loss and cessation of vessel growth.

Studies using animal models of oxygen-induced retinopathy (OIR) have rationalized current ROP treatment and also identified new therapeutic interventions, which may be used to prevent or predict ROP.

PATHOGENESIS OF ROP

What contributes to the susceptibility of the immature retina of the preterm infant and what are the differences between the in utero and extra uterine environment that contribute to the cessation of postnatal retinal vascular growth?

Normal Retinal Development

To understand pathology, we must understand normal retinal vascular development. In the human, retinal vascularization occurs predominantly in the second and third trimesters in utero and reaches maturity at 36 to 40 weeks PMA through vasculogenesis and angiogenesis.[8,16,17] The scaffold of the future retinal vasculature is laid down by vascular precursor cells (vasculogenesis) from 12 weeks to approximately 21 weeks GA, before viable preterm birth.[18,19]

Angiogenesis commences at approximately 17 weeks PMA and expands on the vascular scaffold starting at the optic nerve radiating outward. New vessels bud from existing ones until vascular development is complete, just prior to full-term birth.[19] Angiogenesis is stimulated by the "physiologic hypoxia" of the developing retina described in animal studies.[20] That is, when the metabolic demands of the maturing neural retina outpace the oxygen supplied by the underlying choroid, and the encroaching retinal vascular network, vasoactive factors (particularly vascular endothelial growth factor [VEGF]) are secreted by the avascular retina, which stimulates new vessel formation.[8,20–22]

PHASE I ROP: INTERRUPTION OF DEVELOPMENT WITH HYPEROXIA AND UNDERNUTRITION

Just as the formation of the retinal vasculature responds to "physiologic" hypoxia with developmental progression, it is sensitive to nonphysiologic hyperoxia, which is often encountered after preterm birth. The oxygen saturation of the fetus in the uterine environment is approximately 60% to 70%. Thus preterm birth into room air often causes an increase in oxygen saturation, which is further exacerbated by supplemental oxygen.[23] Hyperoxia suppresses "physiologic hypoxia" causing downregulation of hypoxia-inducible factor regulated growth factors resulting in disruption of normal vascular development.[8,24] Notably, the loss of factors from the maternal fetal interface, (eg, nutrition and other mediators of postnatal growth) also contributes to low serum insulinlike growth factor 1 (IGF-1) and disruption in vessel growth and phase I of ROP.[24]

PHASE II ROP

In severely affected infants, a proliferative phase (phase II) follows the vessel loss of Phase I.[8] The degree of hypoxia and extent of avascular retina induced by phase I ROP determine the degree of hypoxia-derived proliferative factors, which determine the degree of phase II ROP. Phase II begins to develop after more than 32 postmenstrual weeks but can have a wide range of onset.[25,26] Even infants born at 32 weeks GA are susceptible to vessel loss when exposed to very high oxygen saturations after birth resulting in severe proliferative ROP.[27]

The transition to phase II occurs when the attenuated vasculature cannot supply enough oxygen (and nutrients) to the developing retina, leading to increased expression of hypoxia-induced factors. These growth factors then stimulate aberrant vessel formation at the junction between vascularized and avascular retina.[24] Paradoxically these pathologic vessels do not reperfuse the avascular retina but stop at the avascular junction. If the retina receives ample oxygenation, then these pathologic vessels may regress. If the demands of the retina continue to outstrip the oxygen and nutrient supply, then exuberant neovascularization may continue.[8] Neovascular proliferation may cause retinal folds, macular dragging, and cicatricial changes sometimes ultimately causing retinal detachment and blindness (**Fig. 1**).

MOLECULAR MECHANISM OF OXYGEN INFLUENCES ON PHASE I AND II OF ROP
Animal Models of Oxygen-induced Retinopathy

Following the first description of the disease in the earliest studies,[7,28] animal studies have uncovered the molecular mediators of the effects of hyperoxia and hypoxia on retinal vascular development.[23,29,30] Animal models of OIR have been developed in the neonatal kitten, dog, rat, and mouse. The mouse OIR model is currently the most commonly used model as it is reproducible, can be reliably quantified, and can be manipulated genetically (**Fig. 2**).[24,30]

HYPOXIA-INDUCED FACTORS AND ROP: VASCULAR ENDOTHELIAL GROWTH FACTOR

The role of the endothelial cell mitogen and vascular permeability factor VEGF, which plays a critical role in both phase I and phase II ROP, was first described in animal studies of OIR.[21,22,30-37]

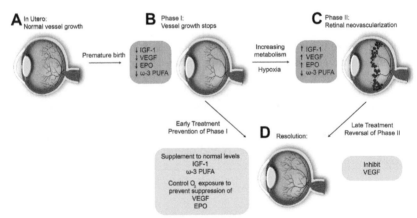

Fig. 1. Treatment of ROP is based on understanding pathogenesis. (1) Laser photocoagulation of ROP: hypoxic retina anterior to neovascularization in phase II of ROP, which produces VEGF, and Epo is destroyed to decrease pathologic blood vessel formation (promoting C to D). (2) Anti-VEGF therapy: direct suppression of neovascularization with suppression of VEGF (promoting C to D). (3) Increasing IGF-1 to in utero levels after birth: prevents vessel loss (phase I) (preventing A to B) to prevent phase II (C). (4) Control of oxygen after preterm birth: prevents hyperoxia-induced suppression of hypoxia-inducible factor–regulated factors VEGF and Epo that are necessary for normal retinal vascular development thus preventing vessel loss (preventing A to B). (5) Maintaining adequate intake of the essential fatty acid DHA after preterm birth: promotes normal vascularization and directly inhibits neovascularization (promote B to D and C to D). (6) Monitoring postnatal growth, which is based on rate of increase of postnatal IGF-1 levels: predicts the future development of neovascular ROP (C).

Room air   75% O$_2$ Room air

P1 $\longrightarrow$ P7 $\longrightarrow$ P12 $\longrightarrow$ P17

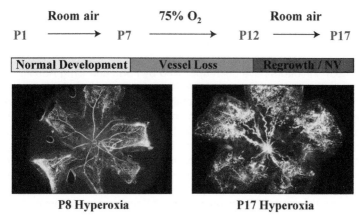

| Normal Development | Vessel Loss | Regrowth / NV |

P8 Hyperoxia   P17 Hyperoxia

Fig. 2. Mouse model of OIR. Neonatal mice are exposed to 75% oxygen from postnatal day 7 (P7) until P12 causing vessel loss and cessation of vascular growth to simulate phase I of ROP. The central retinal microvessels are obliterated and radial vascular growth ceases. When the mice are returned to room air with incompletely vascularized retina, retinal neovascularization is seen, similar to phase II of ROP. Vessel proliferation is maximum at P17 and then regresses, which also occurs in human ROP. These changes can be quantified in retinal flat mounts.

PHASE I: VEGF IS SUPPRESSED BY HYPEROXIA, SUPPRESSING NORMAL VESSEL GROWTH

During retinal development, the wave front of "physiologic hypoxia" resulting from increasing metabolic demand of developing neurons, induces a wave of VEGF, which results in extension of forming vessels. The VEGF wave is suppressed with exposure to hyperoxia, causing cessation of normal vascular development seen in phase I of ROP.[20,29–32,36]

In mouse OIR, after 6 hours exposure to 75% oxygen, both VEGF mRNA and protein levels are suppressed with loss of microvessels and cessation of new vessel formation.[22] This vessel loss can be inhibited by intravitreal injection of VEGF or the VEGFR-1–specific ligand placental growth factor-1.[22,33]

CLINICAL IMPLICATIONS OF VEGF AND PHASE I OF ROP

The finding above demonstrates that oxygen suppression of VEGF during phase I of ROP is a major contributor to vessel loss. These animal studies rationalize the judicious use of oxygen during the early postnatal period where there is incomplete retinal vascularization to minimize VEGF suppression to minimize vessel loss.

PHASE II
VEGF is Overexpressed in Phase II Causing Neovascularization

In the mouse OIR model, with return to room air, the now vasocompromised retina becomes hypoxic, which induces VEGF mRNA and protein expression,[21] which are directly linked to aberrant neovascularization.[21,22,34,35]

Clinical Implications of VEGF in Phase II of Retinopathy

Studies in the OIR model again help us understand the pathogenesis of phase II, showing that neovascularization can be inhibited by targeting VEGF in phase II with intravitreal injections of anti-VEGF compounds including antisense oligodeoxynucleotides, antibodies against VEGF, or small interfering RNA.[34,35,38] These animal studies are the basis of the clinical use of intravitreal injections of anti-VEGF drugs for retinopathy and for age-related macular degeneration (AMD).

Several VEGF inhibitors have been approved by Food and Drug Administration for intraocular injection to treat neovascular AMD and diabetic macular edema including an antibody fragment Lucentis© (ranibizumab). The full anti-VEGF antibody, Avastin© (bevacizumab), is used off label for treatment of these diseases. Although Avastin is neither approved for use in eyes, nor in infants, and intravitreal Avastin injections suppress serum VEGF for weeks in preterm infants,[39] reports of its use is steadily increasing. There are several case reports of the use of these agents with moderate success in severe cases of ROP, which have been refractory to laser treatment[40] or in patients with vitreous bleeding or opaque media unsuitable for laser treatment.[41] In these reports, there was regression of ROP with no adverse systemic or intraocular outcomes reported.

Mintz-Hittner and Kuffel studied the effects of bevacizumab treatment of moderate and severe ROP in eyes that had not previously undergone laser ablation.[42] Twenty-two eyes received intravitreal injection of bevacizumab. The mean follow-up was 48.5 weeks. After a single injection, treatment was considered successful in all eyes. Adverse systemic or intraocular outcomes were not examined.[42]

New Anti-VEGF Studies Needed to Optimize Clinical Care

Just as the optimal balance point must be found with supplemental oxygen enough to prevent brain dysfunction and death but not so much that vascular growth in the eye is suppressed, the balance between sufficient and insufficient VEGF is unknown. In phase I ROP, hyperoxia downregulates VEGF thereby pruning the vascular tree because fewer vessels are needed with high oxygen. However, in the hypoxic phase II there is again a need for more vessels, and VEGF is dramatically upregulated, contributing to aberrant vessel growth.[43]

A large randomized controlled clinical trial is needed to determine the appropriate anti-VEGF agent, the appropriate dosing and timing of treatment, as well as the long-term ocular and systemic outcomes. Although current limited studies appear promising, careful attention must be paid to assess potential long-term ophthalmic and neurologic and other systemic consequences of VEGF inhibitor use in the developing neonate because rapid VEGF-dependent development of vital organs such as brain, lungs, and kidneys normally takes place during the third trimester. Anti-VEGF treatment could compromise this development.

VEGF and Laser Ablation Treatment of ROP

Over the last few decades, treatment with retinal ablation (cryotherapy and laser therapy) during phase II of ROP, have decreased severe vision loss.[44–46] The mechanism of the ablative treatment has been rationalized in terms of animal studies showing that hypoxic retina (that is destroyed by these interventions) is the source of angiogenic factor release that causes vasoproliferation. This was confirmed in an autopsy study showing that laser photocoagulation reduced VEGF expression in ROP-treated retina compared to an untreated fellow eye.[47,48]

Erythropoietin

Erythropoietin (Epo) is a second hypoxia-induced factor, independent of VEGF, which has been shown in *in vitro* and *in vivo* in studies in the OIR mouse to be important in normal retinal angiogenesis in phase I and in neovascularization in phase II of

OIR.[24] *In vitro* Epo is as potent as VEGF in inducing angiogenesis.[49–53] Epo is secreted locally in the retina as well as by the fetal liver and adult kidney to induce erythopoiesis in the bone marrow, apoptosis in neurons and vascular cells, and angiogenesis.[37]

Clinical Implications of Epo Contributing to ROP

During phase II ROP, Epo levels rise concomitant with neovascularization. There is at present no anti-Epo drug to inhibit proliferative retinopathy, although the effect of Epo inhibition in phase II is as great as that of inhibiting VEGF, and development of an anti-Epo drug could be beneficial.[54,55]

In some neonatal intensive care units, anemia in premature infants is treated with the administration of recombinant human Epo (rhEPO).[24,56] In a recent retrospective study of premature babies, rhEPO treatment was found to be a risk factor for the development of threshold ROP requiring photoablative laser.[56] A Cochrane review suggested that in humans, EPO use was associated with an increased risk of ROP (any grade) with a similar trend for ROP stage greater than or equal to 3, although infants were not classified according to PMA.[57]

FACTORS LACKING AFTER PRETERM BIRTH AND ROP
Insulinlike Growth Factor-1

Animal studies have been instrumental in understanding the influence of postnatal factors affecting vascular growth on the development of ROP.[58] Specifically, IGF-1 has been shown to be critical in both phase I and phase II of retinopathy in the OIR model in the mouse.[59,60] IGF-1 is a polypeptide that promotes human fetal growth throughout gestation but particularly in the third trimester, IGF-I levels increase both in the maternal serum and in the fetus.[61] Serum IGF-I levels correlate with weight gain throughout childhood.[62]

In premature infants, the sudden loss of the maternal fetal interaction (eg, loss of nutrients in the setting of increased metabolic demand, loss of placental IGF-1, and other regulating factors) contributes to the dramatic reduction in serum IGF-1 after preterm birth. IGF-1 synthesis in the liver of the fetus/preterm infant is dependent on nutrient supply and level of maturity.[63]

Low serum IGF-1 has been correlated with decreased fetal growth and development.[24,64] Comparison of the longitudinal serum levels of IGF-1 between full-term and preterm babies, show that both groups have a decrease in circulating IGF-I levels after birth. However, full-term infants experience a postnatal surge of IGF-I between day 1 and day 15 of life not seen in preterm infants.[65] The immaturity of the very preterm infant in combination with poorly known nutritional needs precludes proper accretion of nutrients, which will likely reduce IGF-1 secretion and therefore slow down maturation.

Studies in animal models have shown the importance of low IGF-1 to the development of ROP.[24,59,60] Both growth hormone and its mediator for growth, IGF-1, are important in angiogenesis. Genetic defects in the growth hormone/IGF-1 axis result in subnormal vascularization of the retina.[66] In IGF-1 knockout mice, retinal vessel growth is suppressed although VEGF levels are comparable in wild type and IGF-1-/- mice suggesting that VEGF is necessary but not sufficient to promote angiogenesis.[60]

IGF-1 is necessary for maximum VEGF signaling of the Akt and MAP kinase pathway critical for endothelial cell survival and proliferation; this suggests that a minimal level of IGF-1 is required for vascular growth, rationalizing the poor vascular growth seen in phase I in premature infants with ROP. This is supported by the increased growth and decreased ROP after early IGF-1 treatment reported in starving mouse pups subjected to OIR.[67]

IGF-1 is also important in phase II ROP. There is suppressed neovascularization in the OIR growth hormone receptor (and IGF-I)–deficient mouse, which is restored through exogenous administration of IGF-I or an IGF-I receptor antagonist. Again, reduction in IGF-I results in a downregulation of VEGF-mediated MAPK and Akt pathway activation rather than directly affecting VEGF levels.[59,68,69]

These animal studies have uncovered the links between IGF-I and VEGF where IGF-I behaves as a permissive agent in VEGF-mediated angiogenesis. In the premature infant, vessel growth is suppressed with the drop in circulating IGF-1 levels. As the infant grows, the body slowly produces endogenous IGF-1; once a threshold is reached, VEGF-induced neovascularization may ensue.

Clinical Implications: Postnatal IGF-1 Levels and Postnatal Growth Predict ROP

These animal studies have also suggested the importance of using either low serum IGF-1 or the linked parameter of poor postnatal weight gain as a predictor for those infants at highest risk for ROP.[3–5,70–74] They also suggest that IGF-1 replacement might prevent ROP and related complications of premature birth by fostering postnatal growth.[75]

Based on these studies, which gave rise to an understanding of the relationship between IGF-1, postnatal growth, and angiogenesis, a new diagnostic algorithm "Weight IGF-I Neonatal ROP" (WINROP™) was developed in 2006. WINROP uses rate of postnatal weight gain as a reflection of IGF-1 or uses weight gain and IGF-1 levels together as highly predictive markers for those infants at increased risk for development of proliferative ROP. The WINROP algorithm predicts which infants will or will not develop ROP by assessing deviations in the rate of increase in weight and serum IGF-1 of infants who later developed severe ROP from those who developed no or mild ROP using online statistical surveillance (www.winrop.com). In the initial cohort of 79 preterm infants followed longitudinally with weekly postnatal weight and serum IGF-1 measurements, all patients who developed proliferative ROP were identified at least 5 weeks before treatment of severe ROP.[3]

After the initial validations using postnatal changes in both IGF-1 and weight gain,[10] this algorithm has been used since 2009 with postnatal weight gain alone with validation in more than 10,000 infants worldwide. The sensitivity (90%–100%) as well as the specificity (38.7%–81.7%) has varied in different international preterm populations in Sweden, Switzerland, Canada, the US, Brazil, and Mexico[4,70–74] this is considered to be due to the different composition and characteristics of the preterm population in different countries. This tool also helped to determine early which infants are at low risk, thus reducing the number of eye examinations in that population while concentrating observation on those infants at high risk.[4]

With the WINROP algorithm, it has become clear that although treatment may not be warranted until many weeks postnatally, the initial changes in weight gain in the first several weeks of life significantly affect ROP development.[4] Several other algorithms have since been developed that confirm that postnatal weight gain can be used to predict later development of ROP.[76,77]

Omega-3 Long Chain Polyunsaturated Fatty Acids in OIR in Mice

Through mouse OIR studies, the important role of the exogenously (usually diet) derived omega-3 long chain polyunsaturated fatty acid (LCPUFA), docosahexaenoic acid (DHA), in preventing ROP has been elucidated.[24,78,79] In the third trimester, there is a massive transfer of essential fatty acids from mother to fetus, which does not occur after preterm birth.

The principal retinal omega-3 LCPUFA is DHA and the main retinal omega-6 LCPUFA is arachidonic acid. Animal studies have shown that the balance of omega-3 to omega-6 LCPUFA in the retina affects vascular and neuronal survival.[24,78] In extremely preterm infants who are given lipids mainly from intravenous supplementation, which does not contain omega-3 LCPUFAs, there is a deficit of this essential fatty acid, which has been shown to be critical in preventing retinopathy in animal models.

In phase II ROP, there is less avascular retina (and decreased neovascularization) in pups raised on an isocaloric diet with 2% of total fatty acids from omega-3 PUFAs in contrast to a diet enriched in omega-6 PUFAs. This suppression of proliferative ROP occurs through improved regrowth of vessels after vessel loss as well as direct suppression of neovascularization in part through suppression of inflammation.[78] Supplementation with the downstream metabolites of omega-3 PUFAs, including neuroprotectin D1, resolvins D1 and E1, and 4HDHA also prevented neovascularization.[78,79]

Clinical Implication of ROP and DHA

The antineovascular effects of the omega-3 PUFA DHA supplementation are as strong as anti-VEGF therapy in the mouse OIR model, suggesting supplementing oral or parenteral intake of DHA is another potential target to control ROP.[24]

SUMMARY

ROP is a clinically multifactorial process with potentially devastating effects on vision in premature infants. Prevention includes improved oxygen control with avoidance of fluctuations and provision of sufficient nutrition as early as possible. New preventative strategies including IGF-1 replacement and DHA supplementation and possible suppression of the hypoxia-related factor, VEGF, have been identified through insights into the molecular pathogenesis of ROP in animal studies. Any strategy that seeks to modulate the key elements in retinal angiogenesis, must consider their phase-specific effects. Further, the WINROP algorithm and others based on our understanding from mouse studies of IGF-1 and the importance of the related postnatal growth in premature infants at risk for ROP provides a novel method of identifying early those infants at highest risk for ROP, potentially targeting therapy and resources more effectively toward these babies.

ACKNOWLEDGMENTS

AH received support from the Swedish Medical Research Council (grant # 2011-2432), Government grants (#ALFGB-137491), VINNOVA (grant # 2009-00221). LEHS received support from Research to Prevent Blindness Sr. Investigator Award, NEI EY017017, NEI EY022275, NIH P01 HD18655, and the Lowy Medical Foundation.

REFERENCES

1. Wikstrand MH, Hard AL, Niklasson A, et al. Maternal and neonatal factors associated with poor early weight gain and later retinopathy of prematurity. Acta Paediatr 2011;100(12):1528–33.
2. Singer D, Muhlfeld C. Perinatal adaptation in mammals: the impact of metabolic rate. Comp Biochem Physiol A Mol Integr Physiol 2007;148(4):780–4.

3. Lofqvist C, Andersson E, Sigurdsson J, et al. Longitudinal postnatal weight and insulin-like growth factor I measurements in the prediction of retinopathy of prematurity. Arch Ophthalmol 2006;124(12):1711–8.
4. Hellstrom A, Hard AL, Engstrom E, et al. Early weight gain predicts retinopathy in preterm infants: new, simple, efficient approach to screening. Pediatrics 2009; 123(4):e638–45.
5. Lofqvist C, Hansen-Pupp I, Andersson E, et al. Validation of a new retinopathy of prematurity screening method monitoring longitudinal postnatal weight and insulinlike growth factor I. Arch Ophthalmol 2009;127(5):622–7.
6. Terry TL. Extreme prematurity and fibroblastic overgrowth of persistent vascular sheath behind each crystalline lens. Am J Ophthalmol 1942;25:203–4.
7. Patz A, Hoeck LE, De La Cruz E. Studies on the effect of high oxygen administration in retrolental fibroplasia. I. Nursery observations. Am J Ophthalmol 1952; 35(9):1248–53.
8. Ashton N, Ward B, Serpell G. Effect of oxygen on developing retinal vessels with particular reference to the problem of retrolental fibroplasia. Br J Ophthalmol 1954;38(7):397–432.
9. Bolton DP, Cross KW. Further observations on cost of preventing retrolental fibroplasia. Lancet 1974;1(7855):445–8.
10. Stenson B, Brocklehurst P, Tarnow-Mordi W. Increased 36-week survival with high oxygen saturation target in extremely preterm infants. N Engl J Med 2011; 364(17):1680–2.
11. Of Prematurity (STOP-ROP), a randomized, controlled trial. I: primary outcomes. Pediatrics 2000;105(2):295–310.
12. Chen ML, Guo L, Smith LE, et al. High or low oxygen saturation and severe retinopathy of prematurity: a meta-analysis. Pediatrics 2010;125(6):e1483–92.
13. Gilbert C, Muhit M. Twenty years of childhood blindness: what have we learnt? Community Eye Health 2008;21(67):46–7.
14. Gilbert C, Foster A. Childhood blindness in the context of VISION 2020–the right to sight. Bull World Health Organ 2001;79(3):227–32.
15. Gilbert C, Fielder A, Gordillo L, et al. Characteristics of infants with severe retinopathy of prematurity in countries with low, moderate, and high levels of development: implications for screening programs. Pediatrics 2005;115(5):e518–25.
16. Roth AM. Retinal vascular development in premature infants. Am J Ophthalmol 1977;84(5):636–40.
17. Michaelson IC. The mode of development of the vascular system of the retina, with some observations on its significance for certain retinal diseases. Trans Ophthalmol Soc UK 68:137–80.
18. Chan-Ling T, McLeod DS, Hughes S, et al. Astrocyte-endothelial cell relationships during human retinal vascular development. Invest Ophthalmol Vis Sci 2004; 45(6):2020–32.
19. Hughes S, Yang H, Chan-Ling T. Vascularization of the human fetal retina: roles of vasculogenesis and angiogenesis. Invest Ophthalmol Vis Sci 2000;41(5): 1217–28.
20. Chan-Ling T, Gock B, Stone J. The effect of oxygen on vasoformative cell division. Evidence that 'physiological hypoxia' is the stimulus for normal retinal vasculogenesis. Invest Ophthalmol Vis Sci 1995;36(7):1201–14.
21. Pierce EA, Avery RL, Foley ED, et al. Vascular endothelial growth factor/vascular permeability factor expression in a mouse model of retinal neovascularization. Proc Natl Acad Sci U S A 1995;92(3):905–9.

22. Pierce EA, Foley ED, Smith LE. Regulation of vascular endothelial growth factor by oxygen in a model of retinopathy of prematurity. Arch Ophthalmol 1996; 114(10):1219–28.
23. Madan A, Penn JS. Animal models of oxygen-induced retinopathy. Front Biosci 2003;8:d1030–43.
24. Smith LE. Through the eyes of a child: understanding retinopathy through ROP the Friedenwald lecture. Invest Ophthalmol Vis Sci 2008;49(12):5177–82.
25. Good WV, Hardy RJ, Dobson V, et al. The incidence and course of retinopathy of prematurity: findings from the early treatment for retinopathy of prematurity study. Pediatrics 2005;116(1):15–23.
26. Austeng D, Kallen KB, Hellstrom A, et al. Natural history of retinopathy of prematurity in infants born before 27 weeks' gestation in Sweden. Arch Ophthalmol 2010;128(10):1289–94.
27. Shah PK, Narendran V, Kalpana N. Aggressive posterior retinopathy of prematurity in large preterm babies in South India. Arch Dis Child Fetal Neonatal Ed 2012; 97(5):F371–5.
28. Campbell K. Intensive oxygen therapy as a possible cause of retrolental fibroplasia; a clinical approach. Med J Aust 1951;2(2):48–50.
29. Chen J, Smith LE. Retinopathy of prematurity. Angiogenesis 2007;10(2):133–40.
30. Smith LE, Wesolowski E, McLellan A, et al. Oxygen-induced retinopathy in the mouse. Invest Ophthalmol Vis Sci 1994;35(1):101–11.
31. Shweiki D, Itin A, Soffer D, et al. Vascular endothelial growth factor induced by hypoxia may mediate hypoxia-initiated angiogenesis. Nature 1992;359(6398):843–5.
32. Leung DW, Cachianes G, Kuang WJ, et al. Vascular endothelial growth factor is a secreted angiogenic mitogen. Science 1989;246(4935):1306–9.
33. Shih SC, Ju M, Liu N, et al. Selective stimulation of VEGFR-1 prevents oxygen-induced retinal vascular degeneration in retinopathy of prematurity. J Clin Invest 2003;112(1):50–7.
34. Aiello LP, Pierce EA, Foley ED, et al. Suppression of retinal neovascularization in vivo by inhibition of vascular endothelial growth factor (VEGF) using soluble VEGF-receptor chimeric proteins. Proc Natl Acad Sci U S A 1995;92(23): 10457–61.
35. Robinson GS, Pierce EA, Rook SL, et al. Oligodeoxynucleotides inhibit retinal neovascularization in a murine model of proliferative retinopathy. Proc Natl Acad Sci U S A 1996;93(10):4851–6.
36. Stone J, Itin A, Alon T, et al. Development of retinal vasculature is mediated by hypoxia-induced vascular endothelial growth factor (VEGF) expression by neuroglia. J Neurosci 1995;15(7 Pt 1):4738–47.
37. Stone J, Chan-Ling T, Pe'er J, et al. Roles of vascular endothelial growth factor and astrocyte degeneration in the genesis of retinopathy of prematurity. Invest Ophthalmol Vis Sci 1996;37(2):290–9.
38. Jiang J, Xia XB, Xu HZ, et al. Inhibition of retinal neovascularization by gene transfer of small interfering RNA targeting HIF-1alpha and VEGF. J Cell Physiol 2009;218(1):66–74.
39. Sato T, Wada K, Arahori H, et al. Serum Concentrations of Bevacizumab (Avastin) and Vascular Endothelial Growth Factor in Infants With Retinopathy of Prematurity. Am J Ophthalmol 2011;153(2):327–333.e1.
40. Shah PK, Narendran V, Tawansy KA, et al. Intravitreal bevacizumab (Avastin) for post laser anterior segment ischemia in aggressive posterior retinopathy of prematurity. Indian J Ophthalmol 2007;55(1):75–6.

41. Kong L, Mintz-Hittner HA, Penland RL, et al. Intravitreous bevacizumab as anti-vascular endothelial growth factor therapy for retinopathy of prematurity: a morphologic study. Arch Ophthalmol 2008;126(8):1161–3.
42. Mintz-Hittner HA, Kuffel RR Jr. Intravitreal injection of bevacizumab (avastin) for treatment of stage 3 retinopathy of prematurity in zone I or posterior zone II. Retina 2008;28(6):831–8.
43. Weidemann A, Krohne TU, Aguilar E, et al. Astrocyte hypoxic response is essential for pathological but not developmental angiogenesis of the retina. Glia 2010; 58(10):1177–85.
44. Shalev B, Farr AK, Repka MX. Randomized comparison of diode laser photocoagulation versus cryotherapy for threshold retinopathy of prematurity: seven-year outcome. Am J Ophthalmol 2001;132(1):76–80.
45. Multicenter trial of cryotherapy for retinopathy of prematurity: preliminary results. Cryotherapy for Retinopathy of Prematurity Cooperative Group. Pediatrics 1988; 81(5):697–706.
46. Tasman W. Ten-year follow-up from the CRYO-ROP study. Arch Ophthalmol 2001; 119(8):1200–1.
47. Young TL, Anthony DC, Pierce E, et al. Histopathology and vascular endothelial growth factor in untreated and diode laser-treated retinopathy of prematurity. J AAPOS 1997;1(2):105–10.
48. Stefansson E. The therapeutic effects of retinal laser treatment and vitrectomy. A theory based on oxygen and vascular physiology. Acta Ophthalmol Scand 2001; 79(5):435–40.
49. Jaquet K, Krause K, Tawakol-Khodai M, et al. Erythropoietin and VEGF exhibit equal angiogenic potential. Microvasc Res 2002;64(2):326–33.
50. Ribatti D, Vacca A, Roccaro AM, et al. Erythropoietin as an angiogenic factor. Eur J Clin Invest 2003;33(10):891–6.
51. Chen J, Connor KM, Aderman CM, et al. Erythropoietin deficiency decreases vascular stability in mice. J Clin Invest 2008;118(2):526–33.
52. Smith SB, Duplantier J, Dun Y, et al. In vivo protection against retinal neurodegeneration by sigma receptor 1 ligand (+)-pentazocine. Invest Ophthalmol Vis Sci 2008;49(9):4154–61.
53. Chen J, Smith LE. A double-edged sword: erythropoietin eyed in retinopathy of prematurity. J AAPOS 2008;12(3):221–2.
54. Manzoni P, Maestri A, Gomirato G, et al. Erythropoietin as a retinal angiogenic factor. N Engl J Med 2005;353(20):2190–1 [author reply: 1].
55. Chen J, Connor KM, Aderman CM, et al. Suppression of retinal neovascularization by erythropoietin siRNA in a mouse model of proliferative retinopathy. Invest Ophthalmol Vis Sci 2009;50(3):1329–35.
56. Suk KK, Dunbar JA, Liu A, et al. Human recombinant erythropoietin and the incidence of retinopathy of prematurity: a multiple regression model. J AAPOS 2008; 12(3):233–8.
57. Aher SM, Ohlsson A. Early versus late erythropoietin for preventing red blood cell transfusion in preterm and/or low birth weight infants. Cochrane Database Syst Rev 2006;(3):CD004865.
58. Gyllensten LJ, Hellstrom BE. Experimental approach to the pathogenesis of retrolental fibroplasia. I. Changes of the eye induced by exposure of newborn mice to concentrated oxygen. Acta Paediatr Suppl 1954;43(100):131–48.
59. Smith LE, Kopchick JJ, Chen W, et al. Essential role of growth hormone in ischemia-induced retinal neovascularization. Science 1997;276(5319):1706–9.

60. Hellstrom A, Perruzzi C, Ju M, et al. Low IGF-I suppresses VEGF-survival signaling in retinal endothelial cells: direct correlation with clinical retinopathy of prematurity. Proc Natl Acad Sci U S A 2001;98(10):5804–8.
61. Langford K, Nicolaides K, Miell JP. Maternal and fetal insulin-like growth factors and their binding proteins in the second and third trimesters of human pregnancy. Hum Reprod 1998;13(5):1389–93.
62. Ong KK, Langkamp M, Ranke MB, et al. Insulin-like growth factor I concentrations in infancy predict differential gains in body length and adiposity: the Cambridge Baby Growth Study. Am J Clin Nutr 2009;90(1):156–61.
63. Fowden AL. The insulin-like growth factors and feto-placental growth. Placenta 2003;24(8–9):803–12.
64. Lutty GA, Chan-Ling T, Phelps DL, et al. Proceedings of the Third International Symposium on Retinopathy of Prematurity: an update on ROP from the lab to the nursery (November 2003, Anaheim, California). Mol Vis 2006;12:532–80.
65. Lineham JD, Smith RM, Dahlenburg GW, et al. Circulating insulin-like growth factor I levels in newborn premature and full-term infants followed longitudinally. Early Hum Dev 1986;13(1):37–46.
66. Hellstrom A, Carlsson B, Niklasson A, et al. IGF-I is critical for normal vascularization of the human retina. J Clin Endocrinol Metab 2002;87(7):3413–6.
67. Stahl A, Chen J, Sapieha P, et al. Postnatal weight gain modifies severity and functional outcome of oxygen-induced proliferative retinopathy. Am J Pathol 2010;177(6):2715–23.
68. Smith LE, Shen W, Perruzzi C, et al. Regulation of vascular endothelial growth factor-dependent retinal neovascularization by insulin-like growth factor-1 receptor. Nat Med 1999;5(12):1390–5.
69. Lofqvist C, Chen J, Connor KM, et al. IGFBP3 suppresses retinopathy through suppression of oxygen-induced vessel loss and promotion of vascular regrowth. Proc Natl Acad Sci U S A 2007;104(25):10589–94.
70. Wu C, Vanderveen DK, Hellstrom A, et al. Longitudinal postnatal weight measurements for the prediction of retinopathy of prematurity. Arch Ophthalmol 2010; 128(4):443–7.
71. Hard AL, Lofqvist C, Fortes Filho JB, et al. Predicting proliferative retinopathy in a Brazilian population of preterm infants with the screening algorithm WINROP. Arch Ophthalmol 2010;128(11):1432–6.
72. Fluckiger S, Bucher HU, Hellstrom A, et al. The early postnatal weight gain as a predictor of retinopathy of prematurity. Klin Monbl Augenheilkd 2011;228(4): 306–10 [in German].
73. Wu C, Lofqvist C, Smith LE, et al. Importance of early postnatal weight gain for normal retinal angiogenesis in very preterm infants: a multicenter study analyzing weight velocity deviations for the prediction of retinopathy of prematurity. Arch Ophthalmol 2012;130(8):992–9.
74. Zepeda-Romero LC, Hard AL, Gomez-Ruiz LM, et al. Prediction of retinopathy of prematurity using the screening algorithm WINROP in a Mexican population of preterm infants. Arch Ophthalmol 2012;130(6):720–3.
75. Vanhaesebrouck S, Daniels H, Moons L, et al. Oxygen-induced retinopathy in mice: amplification by neonatal IGF-I deficit and attenuation by IGF-I administration. Pediatr Res 2009;65(3):307–10.
76. Binenbaum G, Ying GS, Quinn GE, et al. A clinical prediction model to stratify retinopathy of prematurity risk using postnatal weight gain. Pediatrics 2011;127(3): e607–14.

77. Eckert GU, Fortes Filho JB, Maia M, et al. A predictive score for retinopathy of prematurity in very low birth weight preterm infants. Eye (Lond) 2012;26(3):400–6.
78. Connor KM, SanGiovanni JP, Lofqvist C, et al. Increased dietary intake of omega-3-polyunsaturated fatty acids reduces pathological retinal angiogenesis. Nat Med 2007;13(7):868–73.
79. Sapieha P, Stahl A, Chen J, et al. 5-Lipoxygenase Metabolite 4-HDHA is a mediator of the Antiangiogenic effect of {omega}-3 polyunsaturated fatty acids. Sci Transl Med 2011;3(69):69ra12.

Setting Up and Improving Retinopathy of Prematurity Programs
Interaction of Neonatology, Nursing, and Ophthalmology

Brian A. Darlow, MD, FRCP, FRACP, FRCPCH[a],*,
Clare E. Gilbert, MD, MSc, FRCOphth[b], Ana M. Quiroga, RN, BSN[c,d]

KEYWORDS

- Retinopathy of prematurity • Preterm infant • Neonatal intensive care • Prevention
- Interdisciplinary collaboration • Quality improvement

KEY POINTS

- Retinopathy of prematurity (ROP) programs require collaboration between neonatologists, ophthalmologists, nurses, and allied health personnel, together with parents.
- ROP programs should include measures aimed at both primary and secondary prevention:
  o Primary prevention of ROP involves quality improvement involving obstetric, delivery room, and neonatal care.
  o Secondary prevention of ROP involves agreeing criteria for, and providing the means to achieve, case detection (screening) and treatment.
- ROP programs will have different content and emphasis according to whether the setting is in an economically advanced or developing country.

BACKGROUND

Elsewhere in this issue, Zin and Gole review the current incidence of retinopathy of prematurity (ROP). The highest incidence of severe ROP occurs in 2 settings: the most highly developed countries, where disease needing treatment is largely

[a] Department of Paediatrics, University of Otago Christchurch, PO Box 4345, Christchurch 8140, New Zealand; [b] Department of Clinical Research, London School of Hygiene and Tropical Medicine, Keppel Street, London WC1E 7HT, UK; [c] School of Nursing, Universidad Austral, Av Juan de Garay 125 (C1063ABB), Buenos Aires, Argentina; [d] Argentina and National Program of Infant Blindness Prevention due to Retinopathy of Prematurity, National Ministry of Health, Av 9 de Julio 1925 (C1073ABA), Buenos Aires, Argentina
* Corresponding author.
E-mail address: brian.darlow@otago.ac.nz

Clin Perinatol 40 (2013) 215–227
http://dx.doi.org/10.1016/j.clp.2013.02.006
0095-5108/13/$ – see front matter © 2013 Elsevier Inc. All rights reserved.

restricted to the most premature infants of less than 28 weeks' gestation; and in middle-income and emerging economies, where a mixture of ROP first epidemic pattern (poor or no control of supplemental oxygen) and second epidemic pattern (evolving but uneven care of very preterm infants) is seen, and many infants more mature than 32 weeks' gestation and heavier than 1500 g birth weight are also affected.[1,2] The tragedy of the current "third epidemic" of ROP in developing countries is that we already have the knowledge to prevent much of it, but translating that knowledge into practice remains a challenge. We will only succeed in the latter if there is an environment of collaboration between health professionals of many disciplines and by working together with parents, managers, funders, and policy makers.

The concept of a ROP program will vary according to the setting. However, in every situation there should be 2 main aspects: primary prevention of ROP through better overall care, and secondary prevention through case detection (often called screening), treatment, and follow-up. The ultimate aim will be to reduce the incidence and severity of ROP, and detect and treat cases optimally so that the overall burden of childhood blindness, low vision, and other visual sequelae from ROP is minimized.

PRIMARY PREVENTION OF ROP: DEVELOPED MARKET ECONOMIES

Arguably much of the improvement in outcome from neonatal intensive care for very preterm infants born in developed countries over the last few decades has resulted from major changes in the organization and delivery of care, "big ticket" items that have involved collaboration between funders, managers, and clinicians. Such developments include the establishment of high-risk obstetric units, regionalization of neonatal intensive care, and improved neonatal transport systems.

Neonatal Networks, which became established in the 1980s and 1990s and were built on the success of earlier collaborative studies and population-based cohort studies, have also been a major contributor to improved outcomes.[3,4] A Neonatal Network has been described as "a collaboration of several clinical sites/NICUs where there is a common data set that is used for external audits, observational studies, randomized trials, and quality improvement projects."[4] These latter quality improvement projects have become highly developed in some Networks (Vermont Oxford Network,[5] Pediatrix Medical Group,[6] Canadian Neonatal Network[7]) and epitomize collaboration between doctors, nurses, and allied health disciplines.

One of the notable features in almost all network reports is the wide variation in outcome between units, for both mortality and morbidity, including ROP.[5,8–11] Such differences often remain significant after correcting for key case-mix factors, and could be due to other unidentified differences in case mix, size of neonatal intensive care unit (NICU) in that smaller units are likely to have greater variability over time,[12] differences in case ascertainment,[13–15] and important differences in care practices.[5,11] There is clearly scope to further reduce morbidities across the network. One approach is to focus on outlying units and, for instance, to explore the practices adopted by units that do better on average. This approach might generate hypotheses that could be tested in a randomized controlled trial. However, targeting systemic quality improvement measures, aimed at reducing the incidence of severe ROP in all units down to, for example, the 20th centile rate, would be likely to prevent more cases overall than if the focus is just on the few poorly performing units.[11]

The major morbidities of very preterm infants, intraventricular/periventricular hemorrhage (IVH), bronchopulmonary dysplasia (BPD), necrotizing enterocolitis (NEC), and ROP have been called the "oxygen radical diseases of prematurity" to emphasize a common role for oxidative stress in their pathogenesis.[16] Although more is now understood about the biological and metabolic pathways involved in each disease, it remains the case that measures aimed specifically at reducing the incidence of one type of morbidity will frequently also provide benefits for other outcomes. For example, in a quality improvement project aimed at reducing the incidence of BPD through identifying and implementing potentially better practices, Payne and colleagues[17] not only reduced the incidence of BPD from 37% to 27% but also reduced severe ROP from 12.3% to 9.1%. Schmidt and colleagues,[18] reporting from the CAP trial of caffeine versus placebo for apnea, found that caffeine not only reduced death or disability at 18 to 21 months of age (odds ratio [OR] 0.77, 95% confidence interval [CI] 0.64–0.93) but also reduced the incidence of severe ROP (OR 0.61, 95% CI 0.42–0.89).

The Neonatal Review Group component of the Cochrane collaboration has been very active in summarizing the available evidence, but there remains insufficient evidence to inform practice in many areas.[19] Moreover, there is often a gap between the efficacy of a particular intervention in clinical trials and its effectiveness when implemented in the real world. Closing that gap may be complex, as illustrated by a recent report on improving evidence-based management of neonatal pain.[20] This report emphasizes that interdisciplinary (medical, nursing, allied health) collaboration, and with parents as key stakeholders, was necessary to enable change to occur. Prevention of ROP also inevitably requires a multifaceted approach and a "bundle" of interventions, although there is often mainly a focus on oxygen saturation targeting (reviewed elsewhere in this issue by Stenson and Fleck). Chow and colleagues[21] introduced a practice change in their unit (an oxygen saturation target of 85%–93% compared with the former target of 90%–98%) and reported a reduction in severe ROP from 10% to 2%, with treatment rates falling from 4% to nil. Their practice change involved the introduction of detailed protocols and education aimed at achieving better compliance with the saturation target. The Pediatrix Group, which cares for 25,000 to 30,000 North American very low birth weight infants per annum, introduced a comprehensive oxygen management program, which did not mandate rigid oxygen saturation targets, but was a mix of staff education and measures to achieve better target compliance and to reduce large fluctuations in oxygen saturation.[22] The incidence of severe ROP in the Network decreased from 11% before the program to 5.8% afterward.

PRIMARY PREVENTION OF ROP: MIDDLE-INCOME AND EMERGING ECONOMIES

A decade or more ago, in many of the middle-income and emerging economies experiencing an increase in the incidence of ROP there was often limited awareness of the disease among health funders, health professionals, and the public at large.[2] Attention was drawn to the problem following surveys of children in schools for the blind.[23,24] The control of childhood blindness is a priority of the global initiative to eliminate avoidable blindness, VISION 2020, and with the support of several international agencies and nongovernmental organizations several initiatives have been undertaken to address the problem of ROP from the late 1990s, initially in Latin America.[25] Although the process has differed according to the local requirements and has needed to be driven by local champions (usually ophthalmologists or neonatologists/pediatricians), national and regional workshops on ROP have followed similar patterns and have involved establishing partnerships between institutions, building local capacity and gathering epidemiologic data (**Box 1**).[25] Participants initially were mainly ophthalmologists and neonatologists/pediatricians, but rapidly the need to involve nurses, nurse assistants, and managers was recognized. A major outcome of such workshops

> **Box 1**
> **Outline of national workshops on ROP**
>
> • Establish National ROP working group
>
> • Undertake situational analysis to assess size and demographics of population at risk
>
> • Develop methodology for data collection
>
> • Increase awareness and understanding of ROP and prevention strategies, including need for eye examinations and treatment
>
> • Assess equipment needs (indirect ophthalmoscopes, lasers) and logistics of treatment
>
> • Address training needs, particularly for ophthalmologists
>
> • Develop plans for follow-up of children in pediatric and low-vision clinics
>
> • Increase public awareness and engage with parent organizations
>
> • Advocate with government and health authorities

has been agreed national guidelines on which infants qualify for examination for ROP and the timing of first examinations.[26,27]

Primary prevention of ROP in middle-income countries includes measures aimed at reducing rates of prematurity (now a major focus for the World Health Organization [WHO])[28]; improving antenatal and perinatal care, including access to services and use of antenatal steroids; and improving neonatal care, including care in the delivery room and the crucial first hour of life. Some of these are "big ticket" items while others, such as antenatal steroids, are cheap and easy to administer. Over a decade ago, Higgins and colleagues[29] reported from a retrospective study that receipt of antenatal steroids to the mother significantly decreased the risk of ROP stage 2 or greater. Although not all reports confirm these findings, the benefits from antenatal steroids in terms of reducing mortality and overall morbidity and their safety led the latest Cochrane review to conclude that "a single course of antenatal corticosteroids should be considered routine for preterm delivery with few exceptions."[30] While the delay in uptake of this therapy in developed countries has been well documented[31] and addressed,[32] the low rates of usage in less developed countries has been largely ignored until recently.[33]

Delivery room care of very preterm infants in developed countries has undergone several changes in recent years and has evolved to a "gentler, kinder" approach.[34] This method includes prevention of hypothermia,[35] consideration of delayed cord clamping,[36] minimizing lung damage by avoiding initial 100% oxygen,[37] and early use of nasal continuous positive airway pressure.[38–40] All this requires a team approach but, unfortunately, in many middle-income countries very preterm infants are often born in a hospital distant from the neonatal unit and even when born in the same hospital, neonatal teams (neonatal residents and nurses) rarely attend these deliveries. Primary prevention of ROP through improved neonatal care is also highly feasible in resource-poor settings by adoption of low-cost better practices,[41] including better avoidance and prevention of pain, measures to decrease rates of sepsis,[42] encouraging early receipt of breast milk, improving nutrition, and use of kangaroo care and other supportive care practices.

Underpinning the ability to deliver good-quality care in any setting is the availability of trained nursing staff. The United Kingdom Neonatal Staffing study found that risk-adjusted mortality in their 54 NICUs increased as cot capacity, and therefore nursing workload, increased.[43] Whereas in more developed countries a nurse to patient ratio in intensive care of 1:1 or 1:2 is the norm, in less developed countries there is often a severe shortage of trained nursing staff. Zin and colleagues,[44] in a study from 7 NICUs in Rio de Janeiro, reported that rates of ROP varied from 2.1% to 7.8%. The NICUs with the highest rates of severe ROP also had the poorest nurse to infant ratios of 1:8 and 1:17 (Zin A, personal communication, 2006). In these situations much care is often given by nurse assistants who have very limited training. In the context of the human immunodeficiency virus/AIDS epidemic the WHO recommends that, where appropriate, some tasks can be delegated to less specialized health workers.[45] Although the context is different, through education packages and team building, both nurses and nurse assistants in neonatal care can become empowered to have more responsibility.[41]

Most recent reports from Latin America do suggest that there have been improvements in the prevention of ROP. Until recently Argentina had one of the highest incidences of ROP in Latin America. Guidelines on screening for ROP were published in 1999. In 2003 a Multicenter Collaborative Working Team affiliated to the Ministry of Health was set up with the aim of improving ROP prevention, screening, and treatment. One task was to survey the results of ROP screening and the awareness of ROP. With support from the international charity ORBIS, screening rates were improved, and through the United Nations Children's Fund (UNICEF) the provision of air-oxygen blenders, pulse oximeters, and lasers was increased and educational materials produced. Nurses had a key role in embracing the new technology, increasing the awareness of ROP and leading the changes in clinical practice, including having defined oxygen saturation targets. A recent report from 3 units in Córdoba has documented a decrease in the incidence of type 1 ROP over time.[46]

SECONDARY PREVENTION OF ROP: CASE DETECTION AND TREATMENT

Many industrialized countries of North America, Western Europe, and the Pacific Rim have established guidelines issued by expert bodies concerning which infants should be examined for ROP and when, and on treating ROP. The guidelines should be based on local epidemiology and be regularly reviewed and updated as, for example, has been the case in Sweden[47–49] and the United Kingdom.[50,51] Strictly speaking these are not "screening" programs, which would entail a simple and valid test to identify infants who would then need a gold-standard diagnosis, but rather are "case detection" programs.[2] In the United Kingdom the revised guidelines were drafted jointly by the Royal College of Paediatrics and Child Health, the Royal College of Ophthalmologists, the British Association of Perinatal Medicine, and the premature baby charity BLISS, who represented consumer interests.[51] In the United States the guidelines are a joint statement from the American Academy of Pediatrics, the American Academy of Ophthalmologists, the American Association for Pediatric Ophthalmology and Strabismus, and the American Association of Certified Orthoptists.[52] Both the United Kingdom and United States guidelines give recommendations on which infants to examine and when, criteria for treatment, communication between services and with parents, and a comment on responsibilities for care. Such guidelines will need to be expanded into specific protocols developed through a multidisciplinary consultation process for the needs of every NICU caring for infants who qualify for screening.[53]

An example of all the steps that might be involved in implementing the guidelines is shown in **Fig. 1**. The unit should have agreed written protocols that cover all steps. The simplest method to ensure that all eligible infants are examined at an appropriate time is to identify them when they are first admitted to the NICU by entering their

Infants	Process	Parents
Eligible infants identified at admission (according to local guidelines). Examination date booked	Regular day and time each week for screening	Brief information about ROP in Admission Booklet for parents of babies at risk
ROP coordinator prepares list of infants to be examined. Checks with the neonatal team. Feeding times organized	Location of screening: ideally quiet darkened room in NICU equipped with air/oxygen suction, and resuscitation trolley. Infants on assisted ventilation can be examined in NICU	Reminded of need to examine eyes some time before event: information sheet on screening for ROP. Concerns addressed
Pupil dilatation: local preferences, eg, 2.5% cyclopentolate and 1% phenylephrine $\times$ 2 at 5-minute intervals, 30–60 minutes pre-examination Pain control: local anaesthetic, eg, 0.5%–1% roparacaine. Oral sucrose immediately prior to examination	Equipment: eyelid speculum and scleral indentors; ideal is new sterile set for each case. Indirect ophthalmoscope and 28 diopter lens/wide-field digital imaging system. Sterile gloves. Labeled recording sheet for each baby	Parents told findings (usually by ophthalmologist). More detailed information sheet on ROP and sheet on treatment if necessary. Informed of date of next review
Postexamination monitoring for 24 hours: heart rate and oxygen saturation	Experienced nurse cares for infant during examination. Infant swaddled, heart rate monitor and pulse oximeter attached; consider pacifier	At transfer or discharge parents have a copy of the examination findings and date of next examination or follow-up, and understand the need for these
	Results of each examination and the management decision clearly documented in agreed place in notes	
	Treatment: within 48 hours of treatable disease being detected	

Fig. 1. Outline of ROP screening program.

details into a book or electronic database, and to note and book the date of their first examination at that time. Most units will appoint a nurse ROP coordinator to oversee the program.

Studies have shown that even well-organized systems can break down in several scenarios, such as: when an infant is transferred to another hospital or is discharged home before examinations have been completed; if there is consideration of deferring an examination such as for acute illness in an infant; the ophthalmologist not being available; or if there is a category of discretional examinations such as for very sick infants who do not meet the usual criteria for birth weight or gestational age. Deciding when examinations are complete and organizing timely treatment and further longer-term follow-up also remains a challenge, requiring clear communication between different professional groups, between NICUs and, importantly, with parents (**Box 2**).

Both Australia and New Zealand have published guidelines on which infants to examine, and the Australian and New Zealand Neonatal Network collects perinatal information on high-risk infants in both countries, although data on examinations for ROP are missing for 8% to 10% of infants of less than 29 weeks' gestation.[11] Whether these infants have been examined is unclear. In the United Kingdom, a comprehensive audit of the 1995 national guidelines has been carried out.[54,55] Although most ophthalmologists complied with or exceeded screening guidelines, 7% used criteria that meant not all infants meeting guideline recommendations would be screened, and availability of written information was generally poor.[55] The audit also identified a lack of clarity about responsibilities for ensuring ongoing examinations following transfer or discharge. These issues have all been clearly addressed in the updated 2008 United Kingdom guidelines.[50]

Organizational issues, similar to those in the United Kingdom, have also been identified in the United States.[56] A recent report from the United States, where infants are often discharged home at an earlier stage than in some other countries, has highlighted the problems of completing screening examinations and follow-up after discharge.[57] Parent focus groups and provider interviews were undertaken. Problems with and gaps in care were identified, and solutions suggested. The investigators noted that concerns of ophthalmologists about reimbursement and liability needed to be addressed. Having ophthalmology follow-up services in a multispecialty clinic for very low birth weight children is a suggestion that would be welcomed in other jurisdictions as well, although it may be often difficult to achieve.

In India, Vinekar and colleagues[58] have demonstrated that screening rates can be improved even in poorly resourced areas by low-cost red-alert cards attached to the cots of preterm infants on the day of admission, in this case those with birth weights of 2000 g and less. In several Latin American countries (Argentina, Brazil, Chile, Mexico, Peru) examinations according to local guidelines are now mandatory and, although this still does not always guarantee that every eligible child is examined, it is certainly a strong inducement to ensure that screening does take place.

The recording of the findings at examination is another area where problems can arise, despite the widespread adoption of standard recording forms such as that based on the International Classification of ROP consensus.[59] Trese[60] has described the process as "transcription from the physician's memory to a drawing... [that is] a constant source of controversy in ... malpractice cases." The possible role of photographic images to provide a permanent record of findings at the time of examination is discussed in the article by Wilson and Fielder elsewhere in this issue. Where the results are filed is another issue that needs to be addressed in a consistent way. Lack of readily available records impedes good care at the next examination and follow-up.

Box 2
Screening problems for ROP and possible solutions

Problem	Solution
Transfer to another hospital before eye examination starts or is completed	Clear information on past examinations (if any) and date of next scheduled examination in referral letter. Parents have copy of letter. Consultant neonatologist has responsibility to see that receiving team is aware of this schedule
Discharged home before eye examinations completed	Question whether discharge home at this time is the best strategy. If yes, date and time of next exam confirmed *and* arrangements for family to attend are made. Family contacted again before examination and transport provided if needed
Scheduled eye examination deferred for any reason	Consultant review of decision to defer. If confirmed, state reasons clearly in the medical record. Immediately reschedule examination within 1 week
Discretionary examination for infants outside routine screening criteria	As soon as decision is made to examine, enter details and time of examination in ROP book or electronic system. Inform parents
Deciding when examinations are complete; standard is when the eye fully vascularized or the vessels are well into zone 3	If infant has postmenstrual age less than 37 weeks, a further examination should still be considered even if vessels are into zone 3
Organizing timely treatment	All treatment should be within 48 hours of decision to treat even if that entails transfer elsewhere. Type 1 ROP can progress very rapidly to a worse situation
Organizing follow-up	Time and place of appointment made when decision to follow up is made, and is clearly documented in the main body of the notes and in a letter to all professionals involved in follow-up, of which parents have a copy. Ideally eye appointments should be coordinated with those in other services

Systems are being devised that will allow the findings to be recorded and available electronically. A Web-based Swedish register at present only records the results of screening when the last examination is performed.[61] When they have been involved in care decisions throughout their infant's neonatal course most parents are strong advocates for their child, and providing parents with a copy of the examination record can be a successful strategy.

PARENTS AS PARTNERS IN ROP PROGRAMS

As noted throughout this review, ROP prevention is a team responsibility, and parents must be seen as equal partners in that team. Good communication is at the heart of the relationship between the baby's present medical caregivers and the parents, the future caregivers, which unfolds as neonatal care progresses.[62] Parents should be provided with as much information as they wish and at their pace. Not all parents want all possible information at an early stage or to be involved in all aspects of care,[63]

Box 3
Useful Web sites on ROP for parents

1. http://www.rcpch.ac.uk/system/files/protected/page/ROP%20Guideline%20-%20Jul08%
   20final.pdf
   United Kingdom guidelines, with parent information pamphlets. These guidelines have
   been jointly produced by the Royal College of Ophthalmologists www.rcophth.ac.uk, the
   Royal College of Pediatrics and Child Health www.rcpch.ac.uk, and the British Association of
   Perinatal Medicine www.bapm.org. Has a useful diagram.

2. http://www.nei.nih.gov/health/rop/index.asp
   United States National Eye Institute

3. http://www.aboutkidshealth.ca/En/ResourceCentres/PrematureBabies/
   AboutPrematureBabies/OtherConditions/Pages/Retinopathy-of-Prematurity-ROP.aspx
   Toronto Sick Kids, Canada

4. http://www.healthhaven.com/retinopathy_of_prematurity.htm
   Has mix of sites, many of which are from hospitals or parent organizations and of good
   quality.

5. http://telemedicine.orbis.org/bins/home.asp
   Has good diagrams, which are also available on the Association of Retinopathy and Related
   Diseases (ROPARD) site.

All sites were accessed on December 4, 2012, but be aware that some content may change.

---

although many do. Such information should be, as far as possible, consistent across different members of the team. Having appropriate written information is one way of helping with this consistency, and will assist parents' understanding. Nursing staff inevitably spend most time talking to parents and are often the most trusted members of the team, so their input into the written material and how it is presented is vital.

Examples of information that can be adapted for local use have been published,[62] and there are some excellent Web-based resources (**Box 3**). As well as a mention in an Admission Booklet, many NICUs will have specific written information on ROP, and about screening for ROP and its treatment should the latter be necessary. Before birth or early in the preterm infant's course, ROP will not be a major concern but should be mentioned together with the need for screening. Even in the smallest infants, the prospects for good visual outcomes are excellent. As the time for screening approaches, parents should be reminded of the need to undertake this and be informed as to what will be involved. Parents should be made aware that mild ROP is common and usually resolves spontaneously without adverse consequences. The ophthalmologist, supported by 1 or more familiar members of the team, is best placed to discuss the findings with parents. Caregivers need to be sensitive to the fact that severe ROP may arise at the time the infant is often recovering from most other problems and when parents are beginning to relax.

A complete ROP program must include a plan for follow-up and responsibilities to see that this occurs. Most very preterm infants in need of ophthalmology follow-up will also be being seen in pediatric follow-up clinics, and pediatricians are best placed to oversee the process in partnership with parents.

SUMMARY

This article highlights that all ROP programs should include an emphasis on primary prevention through improved obstetric and neonatal care, and secondary prevention through appropriate case detection and treatment. In less developed countries the first steps might be to raise awareness about ROP and of the potential to reduce the risk of blindness from the disease. Identification of local champions, gathering epidemiologic data, and establishing guidelines for screening and treatment are early steps along the path to a full program. In highly developed countries the variability in outcomes between different units attests to the fact that further improvements are possible through ongoing quality-assurance programs. In all settings the initiation and maintenance of effective programs requires a team approach, with clear and good leadership and a partnership between neonatologists, ophthalmologists, nurses, allied health staff, and parents, together with the support of managers and funders. Even when there are clear and comprehensive guidelines for screening and treatment, there is still the potential for some children to miss an examination at the appropriate time, for treatment to be delayed or even missed, and for follow-up not to occur. Good awareness of these problems, clear-cut organizational responsibilities and, probably most importantly, working closely with parents as equal partners should prevent most of these difficulties.

REFERENCES

1. Gilbert C, Fielder A, Gordillo L, et al. Characteristics of infants with severe retinopathy of prematurity in countries with low, moderate, and high levels of development: implications for screening programs. Pediatrics 2005;115(5):e518–25.
2. Gilbert C. Retinopathy of prematurity: a global perspective of the epidemics, population of babies at risk and implications for control. Early Hum Dev 2008; 84(2):77–82.
3. Thakkar M, O'Shea M. The role of neonatal networks. Semin Fetal Neonatal Med 2006;11(2):105–10.
4. Valls-i-Soler A, Halliday HL, Hummler H. International perspectives: neonatal networking: a European perspective. NeoReviews 2007;8:e275–81.
5. Horbar JD. The Vermont Oxford Network: evidence-based quality improvement for neonatology. Pediatrics 1999;103(1 Suppl E):350–9.
6. Spitzer AR, Ellsbury DL, Handler D, et al. The Pediatrix Babysteps® Data Warehouse and the Pediatrix QualitySteps improvement project system—tools for "meaningful use" in continuous quality improvement. Clin Perinatol 2010;37(1):49–70.
7. Cronin CM, Baker GR, Lee SK, et al. Reflections on knowledge translation in Canadian NICUs using the EPIQ method. Healthc Q 2011;14(Spec No 3):8–16.
8. Horbar JD, Soll RF, Edwards WH. The Vermont Oxford Network: a community of practice. Clin Perinatol 2010;37(1):29–47.
9. Lee SK, McMillan DD, Ohlsson A, et al. Variations in practice and outcomes in the Canadian NICU Network: 1996-1997. Pediatrics 2000;106(5):1070–9.
10. Heuchan AM, Evans N, Henderson-Smart DJ, et al. Perinatal risk factors for major intraventricular haemorrhage in the Australian and New Zealand Neonatal Network, 1995 to 1997. Arch Dis Child 2002;86(2):F86–90.
11. Darlow BA, Hutchinson JL, Simpson JM, et al. Variation in rates of severe retinopathy of prematurity among Neonatal Intensive Care Units in the Australian and New Zealand Neonatal Network. Br J Ophthalmol 2005;89(12):1592–6.
12. Simpson JM, Evans N, Gibberd RW, et al. Analysing differences in clinical outcomes between hospitals. Qual Saf Health Care 2003;12(4):257–62.
13. Walsh MC, Yao Q, Gettner P, et al. Impact of a physiologic definition on bronchopulmonary dysplasia rates. Pediatrics 2004;114(5):1305–11.
14. Harris DL, Bloomfield FH, Teele RL, et al. Variable interpretation of ultrasonograms may contribute to variation in the reported incidence of white matter

damage between newborn intensive care units in New Zealand. Arch Dis Child Fetal Neonatal Ed 2006;91(1):F11–6.

15. Darlow BA, Elder MJ, Horwood LJ, et al. Does observer bias contribute to variations in the rate of retinopathy of prematurity between centres? Clin Experiment Ophthalmol 2008;36(1):43–6.

16. Saugstad O. Oxidative stress in the newborn—a 30-year perspective. Biol Neonate 2005;88(3):228–36.

17. Payne NR, LaCorte M, Karna P, et al. Reduction of bronchopulmonary dysplasia after participation in the Breathsavers Group of the Vermont Oxford Network Neonatal Intensive Care Quality Improvement Collaborative. Pediatrics 2006; 118(Suppl 2):S73–7.

18. Schmidt B, Roberts RS, Davis P, et al. Long-term effects of caffeine therapy for apnea of prematurity. N Engl J Med 2007;357(19):1893–902.

19. Sinclair J. Evidence-based therapy in neonatology: distilling the evidence and applying it in practice. Acta Paediatr 2004;93(9):1146–52.

20. Spence K, Henderson-Smart D. Closing the evidence-practice gap for newborn pain using clinical networks. J Paediatr Child Health 2011;47(3):92–8.

21. Chow LC, Wright KW, Sola A, et al. Can changes in clinical practice decrease the incidence of severe retinopathy of prematurity in very low birth weight infants? Pediatrics 2003;111(2):339–45.

22. Ellsbury DL, Ursprung R. Comprehensive oxygen management for the prevention of retinopathy of prematurity: the Pediatrix experience. Clin Perinatol 2010;37(1): 203–15.

23. Gilbert CE, Rahi J, Eckstein M, et al. Retinopathy of prematurity in middle-income countries. Lancet 1997;350(9070):12–4.

24. Quinn GE, Gilbert C, Darlow BA, et al. Retinopathy of prematurity: an epidemic in the making. Chin Med J (Engl) 2010;123(20):2929–37.

25. Farrell V. Vision 2020 in Latin America. Uniting to fight against retinopathy of prematurity. Ophthalmology Times Europe 2008;4(6). Available at: http://www. oteurope.com/ophthalmologytimeseurope/article/articleDetail.jsp?id=533573. Accessed December 11, 2012.

26. Zin A, de la Fuente Torres MA, Gilbert C, et al. Ophthalmic and neonatal guidelines for ROP screening and treatment in Latin American Countries. 2007. Available at: www.v2020la.org/english/pdf/publications/GuidelinesROP.pdf. Accessed November 29, 2012.

27. Carrion JZ, Fortes Filho JB, Tartarella MB, et al. Prevalence of retinopathy of prematurity in Latin America. Clin Ophthalmol 2011;5:1687–95.

28. March of Dimes, PMNCH, Save the Children, WHO. Born Too Soon: The global action report on Preterm Birth. In: Howson CP, Kinney MV, Lawn JE, editors. Geneva (Switzerland): World Health Organization; 2012.

29. Higgins RD, Mendelsohn AL, DeFeo MJ, et al. Antenatal dexamethasone and decreased severity of retinopathy of prematurity. Arch Ophthalmol 1998;116(5):601–5.

30. Roberts D, Dalziel S. Antenatal corticosteroids for accelerating fetal lung maturation for women at risk of preterm birth. Cochrane Database Syst Rev 2006;(3):CD004454.

31. Sinclair JC. Meta-analysis of randomized controlled trials of antenatal corticosteroids for the prevention of respiratory distress syndrome: discussion. Am J Obstet Gynecol 1995;173(1):335–44.

32. NIH Consensus Development Panel on the Effect of Corticosteroids for Fetal Maturation on Perinatal Outcomes. Effect of corticosteroids for fetal maturation on perinatal outcomes. JAMA 1995;273(5):413–8.

33. Althabe F, Belizán JM, Mazzoni A, et al. Antenatal corticosteroids trial in preterm births to increase neonatal survival in developing countries: study protocol. Reprod Health 2012;9:22. http://dx.doi.org/10.1186/1742-4755-9-22.

34. Vento M, Cheung PY, Aguar M. The first golden minutes of the extremely-low-gestational-age neonate: a gentle approach. Neonatology 2009;95(4):286–98.

35. McCall EM, Alderdice FA, Halliday HL, et al. Interventions to prevent hypothermia at birth in preterm and/or low birthweight infants. Cochrane Database Syst Rev 2008;(1):CD004210.

36. Rabe H, Diaz-Rossello JL, Duley L, et al. Effect of timing of umbilical cord clamping and other strategies to influence placental transfusion at preterm birth on maternal and infant outcomes. Cochrane Database Syst Rev 2012;(8):CD003248.

37. Perlman JM, Wyllie J, Kattwinkel J, et al. Neonatal resuscitation: 2010 international consensus on cardiopulmonary resuscitation and emergency cardiovascular care science with treatment recommendations. Circulation 2010; 122(16 Suppl 2):S516–38.

38. Morley CJ, Davis PG, Doyle LW, et al. Nasal CPAP or intubation at birth for very preterm infants. N Engl J Med 2008;358(7):700–8.

39. Finer N, Carlo WA, Walsh MC, et al. Early CPAP versus surfactant in extremely preterm infants. N Engl J Med 2010;362(23):1970–9.

40. Dunn MS, Kaempf J, de Klerk A, et al. Randomized trial comparing 3 approaches to the initial respiratory management of preterm neonates. Pediatrics 2011; 128(5):e1069–76.

41. Darlow BA, Zin A, Beecroft G, et al. Capacity building in Rio de Janeiro: methods of the POINTS of Care project to enhance nursing education and reduce adverse neonatal outcomes. BMC Nurs 2012;11:3.

42. Darmstadt GL, Nawshad Uddin Ahmed AS, Saha SK, et al. Infection control practices reduce nosocomial infections and mortality in preterm infants in Bangladesh. J Perinatol 2005;25(5):331–5.

43. Tucker J, UK Neonatal Staffing Study Group. Patient volume, staffing, and workload in relation to risk-adjusted outcomes in a random stratified sample of UK neonatal intensive care units: a prospective evaluation. Lancet 2002;359(9301): 99–107.

44. Zin A, Moreira ME, Bunce C, et al. Retinopathy of prematurity in 7 neonatal units in Rio de Janeiro: screening criteria and workload implications. Pediatrics 2010; 126(2):e410–7.

45. World Health Organization. Taking stock: task shifting to tackle health worker shortages. 2007. Available: http://www.who.int/healthsystems/task_shifting/TTR_tackle.pdf. Accessed December 4, 2012.

46. Urets-Zavalia JA, Crim N, Knoll EG, et al. Impact of changing oxygenation policies on retinopathy of prematurity in a neonatal unit in Argentina. Br J Ophthalmol 2012;96(12):1456–61.

47. Holmström G, el Azazi M, Jacobson L, et al. A population-based, prospective study of the development of ROP in prematurely born children in the Stockholm area of Sweden. Br J Ophthalmol 1993;77(7):417–23.

48. Larsson E, Holmström GS. Screening for retinopathy of prematurity: evaluation and modification of guidelines. Br J Ophthalmol 2002;86(12):1399–402.

49. Austeng D, Källen KB, Hellström A, et al. Screening for retinopathy of prematurity in infants born before 27 weeks' gestation in Sweden. Arch Ophthalmol 2011; 129(2):167–72.

50. Wilkinson AR, Haines L, Head K, et al. UK retinopathy of prematurity guideline. Early Hum Dev 2008;84(2):71–4 (and in Eye 2009;23:2137–9).

51. UK Retinopathy of prematurity guideline May 2008. Available at: http://www. rcophth.ac.uk/page.asp?section=451&sectionTitle=Clinical+Guidelines. Acce ssed November 29, 2012.

52. Fierson WM, American Academy of Pediatrics Section on Ophthalmology, American Academy of Ophthalmology, et al. Screening examination of premature infants for retinopathy of prematurity. Pediatrics 2013;131(1):189–95.

53. VanStone W. Retinopathy of prematurity: an example of a successful screening programme. Neonatal Netw 2010;29(1):15–21.

54. Haines L, Fielder AR, Scrivener R, et al. Retinopathy of prematurity in the UK I: the organisation of services for screening and treatment. Eye 2002;16(1):33–8.

55. Fielder AR, Haines L, Scrivener R, et al. Retinopathy of prematurity in the UK II: audit of national guidelines for screening and treatment. Eye 2002;16(3):285–91.

56. Kemper AR, Wallace DK. Neonatologists' practices and experiences in arranging retinopathy of prematurity screening services. Pediatrics 2007;120(3):527–31.

57. Wang CJ, Little AA, Kamholz K, et al. Improving preterm ophthalmologic care in the era of Accountable Care Organizations. Arch Ophthalmol 2012. http://dx.doi.org/ 10.1001/archophthalmol.2012.1890.

58. Vinekar A, Avadhani K, Dogra M, et al. A novel, low-cost method of enrolling infants at risk for retinopathy of prematurity in centres with no screening program: the REDROP study. Ophthalmic Epidemiol 2012;19(5):317–21.

59. International Committee for the Classification of Retinopathy of Prematurity. The international classification of retinopathy of prematurity revisited. Arch Ophthalmol 2005;123(7):991–9.

60. Trese M. What is the real gold standard for ROP screening? Retina 2008; 28(Suppl 3):S1–2.

61. Holmström GE, Hellström A, Jakobsson PG, et al. Swedish national register for retinopathy of prematurity (SWEDROP) and the evaluation of screening in Sweden. Arch Ophthalmol 2012;130(11):1418–24.

62. Darlow BA. Parents and ROP. In: Azad R, Trese MT, editors. Textbook of retinopathy of prematurity. New Delhi: Wolters Kluwer (India); 2011. Chapter 14. p. 195–207. [ISBN: 9788184731996].

63. Janvier A. I'm only punching in. Arch Pediatr Adolesc Med 2007;161(9):827.

Retinopathy of Prematurity and the Oxygen Conundrum
Lessons Learned from Recent Randomized Trials

Brian W. Fleck, MD, FRCOph[a],*, Ben J. Stenson, MD[b]

KEYWORDS

- Oxygen supplementation • Retinopathy of prematurity • Preterm infants
- Neonatal Oxygenation Prospective Meta-analysis (NeoPROM) collaboration

KEY POINTS

- Retinopathy of prematurity (ROP) was first recognized as oxygen supplementation was introduced into neonatal care in the 1940s.
- Oxygen was quickly recognized to have an important role in the causal chain.
- Randomized controlled trials have consistently shown that restricting oxygen results in a lower incidence of severe ROP but at a cost of increased mortality.
- Present evidence suggests that it is unwise to target oxygen-saturation values less than 90% in preterm infants born before 28 weeks' gestation.
- Implementing this evidence is likely to result in a small increase in severe ROP.
- New approaches to the prevention of ROP are required.

HISTORICAL BACKGROUND

When Joseph Priestly first described oxygen more than 200 years ago he raised caution about possible toxicity, commenting that, if breathed by a healthy person, it may cause them to live out too fast. Oxygen rapidly came into use in the care of preterm infants in the 1940s. Seventy years later, the optimal balance of administration to avoid the consequences of both hyperoxia and hypoxia remains unknown.

Terry[1] first described retrolental fibroplasia (RLF), now known as retinopathy of prematurity (ROP), in 1942. Campbell[2] suggested a link with oxygen treatment in 1951. Patz and colleagues[3] published a small clinical trial 1952, which showed that higher levels of inspired oxygen were associated with a higher risk of cicatricial RLF. Ashton[4,5] showed toxic effects of oxygen on retinal blood vessel development in a kitten model. His work further emphasized the toxic effects of oxygen on developing

[a] Department of Ophthalmology, Princess Alexandra Eye Pavilion, Chalmers Street, Edinburgh, EH3 9HA, UK; [b] Neonatal Unit, Simpson Centre for Reproductive Health, Royal Infirmary of Edinburgh, Edinburgh, EH16 4SA, UK
* Corresponding author.
E-mail address: Brian.Fleck@ed.ac.uk

Clin Perinatol 40 (2013) 229–240
http://dx.doi.org/10.1016/j.clp.2013.02.010
0095-5108/13/$ – see front matter © 2013 Elsevier Inc. All rights reserved.

retinal blood vessels, and he recommended that "only the minimal amount consistent with the infant's survival" should be used.

Askie and colleagues[6] summarized the results of oxygen trials in preterm infants in the 1950s in a Cochrane Review. The largest study was published in 1956: the cooperative study of retrolental fibroplasia and the use of oxygen. Reduced (curtailed) oxygen therapy resulted in a lower incidence of RLF than giving 50% oxygen for 28 days of postnatal (routine) oxygen therapy, which was the standard of care at that time.[7] Both vascular RLF and cicatricial RLF occurred more frequently in the routine-oxygen-therapy group. The power calculation for the study was based on the incidence of RLF, not on mortality, and no significant difference in mortality was found between the groups.

INCREASED MORTALITY AND MORBIDITY WITH OXYGEN RESTRICTION

Following publication of the cooperative study, a policy of restricted oxygen therapy was universally adopted. It was anticipated that RLF could be prevented by this approach.[8] However, an excess mortality among preterm infants on the first day of life was clearly shown by Cross[9] using epidemiologic data in 1973. It was estimated that for every case of blindness prevented, 16 infants died.[9] The optimal level of oxygen therapy was unknown, and Cross[9] called for increased resources for the intensive care of preterm infants.

ARTERIAL BLOOD GASES AND TARGET RANGES FOR Po_2

In the 1960s and 1970s it became possible to measure arterial Po_2 by sampling blood from umbilical arterial catheters and thus to titrate oxygen against intermittent measurements of Po_2. Initial practice was to aim for the Po_2 of healthy older individuals. Observational data did not link the development of ROP to exposure to any particular Po_2 level,[10,11] but prospective trials of different Po_2 target ranges were not performed. The introduction of transcutaneous Po_2 electrodes enabled oxygen to be titrated against Po_2 continuously rather than against infrequent blood samples. Bancalari and colleagues[12] asked whether using continuous monitoring of transcutaneous oxygen tension ($TcPo_2$) would reduce the incidence and/or severity of ROP. The target range for Po_2 was 50 to 70 mm Hg (6.7–9.3 kPa). The overall incidence of retinopathy was 51% in the transcutaneous group versus 59% in the standard-care group. Mortality was 32% in the continuous-monitoring group versus 24% in the standard-care group. Neither difference was statistically significant. With an 8% absolute reduction in ROP associated with continuous monitoring but also an 8% increase in mortality, it is regrettable that the trial was not larger because, with the benefit of hindsight, 25 years ahead of the recent trials, this study may represent the first evidence from the era of targeted oxygen therapy that more stringent control of oxygen against measures of oxygenation reduces ROP but at a cost of increased mortality. In a post-hoc analysis of the $TcPo_2$ levels during oxygen therapy in the infants in the continuous-monitoring group, there was a statistically significant relationship between time spent with $TcPo_2$ greater than 80 mm Hg (10.6 kPa) and the incidence and severity of ROP.[13] It became increasingly common practice to target a Po_2 range of 50 to 80 mm Hg and this was recommended in clinical guidelines.[14]

OXYGEN-SATURATION MONITORING

From the 1990s, oxygen-saturation (Spo_2) monitoring became increasingly popular as the main guide to supplemental oxygen administration in neonatal units, which was an important change in approach. Po_2 and Spo_2 are not linearly related, and the many factors influencing hemoglobin/oxygen affinity mean that the Po_2 associated with a given Spo_2 varies within and between infants. As a result, target Po_2 ranges cannot readily be converted to target Spo_2 ranges. Trials were not done to determine whether this move to Spo_2 monitoring would be associated with improved clinical outcomes compared with $TcPo_2$ monitoring or to determine the optimal Spo_2 range to target. In a randomized crossover study in preterm infants comparing transcutaneous $TcPo_2$ monitoring with saturation Spo_2 monitoring, oxygenation was more variable while using Spo_2 than when using $TcPo_2$.[15] A case control cohort study had previously shown that $TcPo_2$ oxygen variability during the first 2 weeks of life was associated with an increased risk of severe ROP.[16] Clinical practice in terms of Spo_2 target range varied widely between neonatal units.[17,18] In the absence of high-quality evidence defining the boundaries, clinicians were attempting to steer a middle way between possible complications of hyperoxia and of hypoxia. Most current research now relates the risks and benefits of different approaches to oxygen administration to measures of Spo_2.

PATHOGENESIS OF ROP: UNDERSTANDING THE EFFECTS OF OXYGEN SUPPLEMENTATION DURING THE TWO PHASES OF ROP DEVELOPMENT

In the past, the pathogenesis of RLF was understood in terms of the clinical oxygen supplementation regimens used in the early 1950s. Several weeks' exposure to high concentrations of inspired oxygen was followed by a rapid return to room air.[3] In a kitten model, this resulted in a vaso-obliteration phase during exposure to high concentrations of oxygen, and a vasoproliferation phase on return to room air.[5] However, understanding of the two phases of ROP development has altered with progress in clinical practice and with the development of better experimental models.

Human retinal blood vessel development normally occurs in a hypoxic environment in utero. The concept of physiologic hypoxia–driven, vascular endothelial growth factor (VEGF)–mediated angiogenesis[19] is central to the current understanding of early postnatal retinal blood vessel development in premature infants.[20] Preterm birth results in higher blood and tissue oxygen levels, which are further increased by oxygen supplementation. Physiologic hypoxia is reduced and retinal vascularization is delayed. In addition, serum levels of insulin like growth factor 1 (IGF1) are low at this time.[21] IGF1 facilitates VEGF signaling,[22] and low serum levels of IGF1 contribute to delayed retinal vascularization: phase 1 of ROP development.[20] Clinical studies of oxygen therapy started soon after birth and continued during the first few weeks of postnatal life investigate this phase of ROP development.

Phase 2 of ROP development occurs when normal angiogenesis is overtaken by pathologic angiogenesis. The peripheral avascular retina continues to grow, and VEGF secretion into the vitreous increases. At the same time, serum IGF1 levels increase,[21] facilitating the effects of VEGF on retinal angiogenesis.[22] Abnormal blood vessels grow out of the retina, toward the high concentrations of VEGF in the vitreous. Extraretinal growth of vascular tissue is termed stage 3 ROP. It has been postulated that increased oxygen supplementation may be beneficial during phase 2 of ROP development: increased tissue oxygen may reduce VEGF levels and arrest progression to severe ROP. Clinical studies of oxygen therapy performed during this phase, typically after 32 weeks gestational age, may be expected to produce different effects on retinal blood vessel development than studies performed in the earlier postnatal period.

THE SUPPLEMENTAL THERAPEUTIC OXYGEN FOR PRETHRESHOLD RETINOPATHY OF PREMATURITY TRIAL

The concept that relative hypoxia in the peripheral avascular retina is responsible for the pathologic angiogenic response in the second phase of ROP, and that this response might be mitigated by increased supplemental oxygen, was tested in the Supplemental Therapeutic Oxygen for Prethreshold Retinopathy of Prematurity (STOP-ROP) trial, published in 2000.[23] This trial differed from other oxygen trials in that it was designed to test a possible treatment of acute, severe ROP, rather than to prevent the development of severe ROP.

Infants with prethreshold ROP in at least 1 eye, who had an oxygen saturation less than 94% in room air, were randomized at a mean postmenstrual age of around 35 weeks to oxygen therapy that resulted in 89% to 95% saturation (conventional oxygen), or 96% to 99% saturation (supplemental oxygen). Forty-eight percent of infants on conventional oxygen and 41% of infants on supplemental oxygen progressed to threshold ROP. After adjustment for baseline factors, there was no significant difference between the groups. At 3 months after term, there was no difference in the structural outcome of the retina (4.8% abnormal in the conventional group and 4.1% in the supplemental group). The supplemental-oxygen group had worse systemic outcomes, with pneumonia or worsening chronic lung disease in 13.2% versus 8.5% in the conventional-oxygen group.

COHORT STUDIES OF REDUCED-OXYGEN THERAPY

Several cohort studies published during the 2000s pointed toward reduced-oxygen treatment producing fewer cases of severe ROP.[17,18,24] Chow and colleagues[24] described a single-center historical comparison, with reduced severe ROP following the adoption of a policy of reduced and more stable oxygen therapy. Tin and colleagues[17] measured the rate of severe ROP in several treatment centers that used differing oxygen therapy policies. They found an association between reduced rates of severe ROP and the use of low-oxygen-saturation protocols. There was no identifiable increase in other morbidities or mortality with lower Spo_2 targets. Anderson and colleagues[18] reported a survey of 142 neonatal treatment centers in North America. Again, there was an association between reduced rates of severe ROP and the use of low-oxygen-saturation protocols.

THE BENEFITS OF OXYGEN SATURATION TARGETING STUDY

The Benefits of Oxygen Saturation Targeting (BOOST) study[25] was performed in Australia, and was published in 2003. The hypothesis behind the study was that chronic hypoxemia in preterm neonates would result in poor growth and development. The power calculation for the study was based on postnatal weight gain and the rate of major developmental abnormality at 12 months of age. Infants born at less than 30 weeks' gestation, who remained oxygen dependent at 32 weeks postmenstrual age, were randomized to standard-saturation oxygen therapy to maintain Spo_2 in the range of 91% to 94%, or high-saturation oxygen therapy with Spo_2 in the range of 95% to 98%. A major innovation in the trial design was the use of specially modified Nellcor N-3000 oximeters that had been internally offset by the manufacturers to read 2% higher or 2% lower than the true Spo_2 so that the intervention could be properly masked, which meant that, if caregivers used an allocated trial oximeter to target the displayed Spo_2 range of 93% to 96%, the patient would have an actual target range of either 91% to 94% or 95% to 98%. Spo_2 data were downloaded from the trial oximeters to measure the actual achieved Spo_2 ranges of the two groups and this was plotted in the form of pooled frequency distributions, as shown in **Fig. 1.** The study methodology resulted in different Spo_2 distributions between the two randomization groups.

The study found no significant differences in the primary outcomes of growth or major developmental abnormality at corrected age 12 months. There was no significant difference in the rates of ROP, of any stage, between the two groups. There was no significant difference in the proportion of infants who needed treatment of acute ROP in the two groups: 20/178 (11%) in the standard-saturation group and 11/180 (6%) in the high-saturation group ($P = .09$). All infants treated for ROP had a gestational age at birth of less than 28 weeks. The proportions of infants of gestational age at birth of less than 28 weeks who needed treatment of acute ROP was 20/124 (16%) in the standard-saturation group, and 11/132 (8%) in the high-saturation group ($P = .06$).

The timing of oxygen therapy intervention is important when interpreting the results of the first BOOST trial. The oxygen interventions were started at 32 weeks' gestation, consistent with the timing of phase 2 of ROP development. This timing may account for the (nonsignificant) reduction of severe ROP in the high-oxygen-saturation group, as also occurred in the STOP-ROP trial.

NEONATAL OXYGENATION PROSPECTIVE META-ANALYSIS COLLABORATION

Following completion of the first BOOST trial, it was recognized that, although individual oxygen treatment trials could show moderate to large differences in mortality and morbidity between groups, a large number of subjects is needed to show a smaller, but clinically significant, difference in mortality or severe disability.[26] A sample size of 5000 infants is needed to detect a 4% difference in death or severe disability.[26] A collaboration of 5 national multicentre randomized controlled trials was formed (**Box 1**), with harmonized study protocols and advance agreement to perform a meta-analysis of the studies.[26] The opposing concerns to be studied were that infants exposed to lower levels of oxygen (<90% saturation) during the first few weeks of life

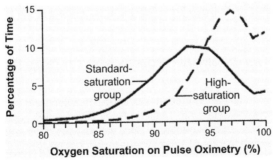

Fig. 1. Pooled frequency distribution curves of time spent at each oxygen saturation in the two groups in the first BOOST trial. The saturation values were sampled every 10 seconds during intermittent downloads performed approximately twice weekly and lasting 8–24 hours each. The median oxygen saturation was 93% in the standard-saturation group (interquartile range, 90%–96%) and 97% in the high-saturation group (interquartile range, 94%–98%). (*From* Askie LM, Henderson-Smart DJ, Irwig L, et al. Oxygen-saturation targets and outcomes in extremely preterm infants. N Engl J Med 2003;349(10):963; with permission. Copyright © 2003, Massachusetts Medical Society.)

Box 1		
Trials include in the NeoPROM prospective meta-analysis collaboration		
Name of Trial	**Country**	**Planned Sample Size**
Surfactant, Positive Pressure, and Oxygenation Randomized Trial (SUPPORT)	United States	1310
BOOST II	Australia	1200
BOOST II	New Zealand	320
BOOST II	United Kingdom	1200
Canadian Oxygen Trial (COT)	Canada	1200

may be at greater risk of death, cerebral palsy, patent ductus arteriosus (PDA), pulmonary vascular resistance, and apnoea,[27–29] whereas infants exposed to higher levels of oxygen (>90% saturation) may be at greater risk of ROP[17,18,24] and chronic lung disease. The (negative) hypothesis of the Neonatal Oxygenation Prospective Meta-analysis (NeoPROM) collaborative meta-analysis is that, compared with a target range for Spo_2 of 91% to 95%, targeting Spo_2 of 85% to 89% within 24 hours of birth until 36 weeks postmenstrual age is associated with less than 4% absolute risk difference in mortality and major disability by 2 years of age.

As in the first BOOST study, the 5 NeoPROM trials used specially offset oximeters to mask the intervention. Masimo Radical oximeters were modified by the manufacturers so that, within the Spo_2 range 85% to 95% they displayed a reading that was either 3% higher or 3% lower than the monitored reading. By targeting a range of 88% to 92%, infants cared for with trial oximeters would thus be targeted to a range of either 85% to 89% or 91% to 95%. Outside the range of 85% to 95%, the oximeters transitioned gradually back to an unmodified reading. Infants born before 28 weeks' gestation were included and the allocated treatment was commenced within 24 hours of delivery. The study interventions were continued until 36 weeks gestational age.

The prospective meta-analysis of data from these 5 trials will take place once each individual trial has reported its primary outcome data. At this time, all of the trials have stopped recruiting infants. Follow-up has been completed in the Surfactant, Positive Pressure, and Oxygenation Randomized Trial (SUPPORT), the New Zealand BOOST II trial, and the Canadian Oxygen Trial (COT) and is ongoing in the UK and Australian BOOST II trials.

NEOPROM TRIALS: AN UNFORESEEN PROBLEM WITH THE OXIMETER CALIBRATION ALGORITHM

After the NeoPROM trials had started, it was shown in a separate investigation by the UK trial investigators that standard Masimo Radical oximeters returned fewer Spo_2 values from 87% to 90% than expected.[30] Spo_2 values were downloaded from the oximeters used in the routine care of 176 oxygen-dependent preterm infant in 35 UK and Irish Neonatal Units. The downloaded Spo_2 data were pooled and plotted as a frequency histogram similar to that published in the first BOOST trial. There was a dip in the histogram, with fewer values than were expected in the Spo_2 range of 87% to 90% (**Fig. 2**).

Because this could affect the lower and higher Spo_2 randomization groups in the oxygen trials differently and might therefore affect the trial results, it was investigated further with assistance from Masimo. A systematic shift up in the oximeter calibration curve between 87% and 90% reduced the frequency of displayed Spo_2 values

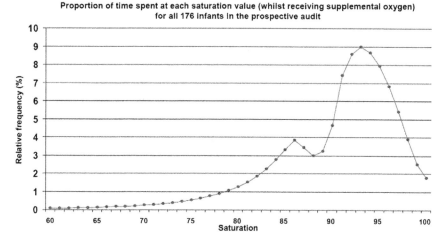

Fig. 2. Pooled frequency distribution curve of time spent at each oxygen saturation while receiving supplemental oxygen in 176 oxygen-dependent preterm infants monitored using standard Masimo Radical oximeters. CI, confidence interval. (*From* Johnston ED, Boyle B, Juszczak E, et al. Oxygen targeting in preterm infants using the Masimo SET Radical pulse oximeter. Arch Dis Child Fetal Neonatal Ed 2011;96:F430; with permission.)

between 87% and 90% and caused SpO_2 values more than 87% to read up to 2% higher, with this increase maximal at an SpO_2 of 90% and becoming smaller at higher values such that it disappeared at SpO_2 values more than 96%. The shift up in the calibration curve has the effect of narrowing the available target range of the lower target group but not the high target group. An increase of the SPO_2 values in the high target group means that their actual values were lower, effectively narrowing the difference between groups.

Masimo supplied software with a revised calibration algorithm that eliminated the unwanted effect and, in direct within-patient comparisons in oxygen-dependent preterm infants, this performed similarly to commonly used oximeters from other manufacturers.[30] The revised calibration algorithm was installed into the trial oximeters in the UK and Australian BOOST II trials between December 2008 and May 2009 and all infants recruited after this time were managed with the revised oximeters. Investigation of the SpO_2 patterns of infants recruited to the trials before and after the change showed that the SpO_2 distributions of the infants were affected by the change and that clearer separation of saturation patterns between the randomization groups was achieved with the new oximeter calibration algorithm than with the original oximeters. It was considered that results obtained with the revised oximeters were likely to be more generalizable.

NEOPROM TRIALS: INITIAL RESULTS FROM THE SUPPORT TRIAL

SUPPORT was the first NeoPROM trial to complete recruitment and report hospital discharge outcomes.[31] The study recruited 1316 infants.[31] A two-by-two factorial design was used; testing 2 forms of ventilation (surfactant with ventilation vs continuous positive airway pressure), and 2 oxygen therapy saturation ranges (85%–89% vs 91%–95%).

The primary composite outcome for the short-term analysis of the oxygen component of the study was severe retinopathy or death before 36 weeks' gestation, although this was changed to severe retinopathy or death before hospital discharge before the initial analysis of the study was performed.[31] Severe retinopathy was defined as ROP that required ophthalmic treatment intervention. There was no significant difference between the groups for the primary composite outcome. However, 130 of 654 (19.9%) infants in the lower-oxygen-saturation group died before hospital discharge, compared with 107 of 662 (16.2%) infants in the higher-oxygen-saturation group (relative risk for lower saturation 1.27, 95% confidence interval [CI] 1.01–1.60, $P = .04$). The rate of severe retinopathy was lower in the lower-oxygen-saturation group (8.6% vs 17.9%, relative risk for lower saturation 0.52, 95% CI 0.37–0.73, $P<.001$). The published report recommended that caution should be exercised regarding a strategy of targeting oxygen-saturation levels in the low range for preterm infants because it may lead to increased mortality. These data were published while the other oxygen trials were still recruiting.

NEOPROM TRIALS: EARLY TERMINATION OF THE UK AND THE AUSTRALIAN TRIALS

In December 2010, the Data Monitoring Committees (DMCs) of the UK and Australian and New Zealand BOOST II trials undertook a joint interim safety analysis, pooling interim data from the 3 trials and considering them alongside the published data from the SUPPORT trial.[32] The sole outcome considered was survival to 36 weeks' gestation. The analysis considered data from 2315 infants in the UK and Australian and New Zealand BOOST II trials, plus 1316 infants in the SUPPORT trial. There were data for 1055 infants recruited to the UK and Australian trials after the revision of the oximeters. Guidelines for the analysis prespecified that the trial investigators would only be unblinded to the results if a difference in survival between groups for all infants, or for the infants treated using the new oximeters, exceeded 3 standard errors (equivalent to 99.73% CIs, or a P value $<.003$). Results of the analysis are shown in **Fig. 3.**

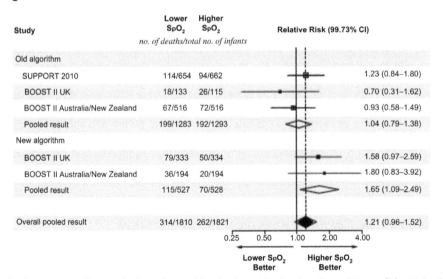

Fig. 3. Interim safety analysis performed by the Data Monitoring Committees of the United Kingdom, Australian, and New Zealand BOOST II trials, which included data from the SUPPORT study. (*From* Stenson B, Brocklehurst P, Tarnow-Mordi W, et al. Increased 36-week survival with high oxygen saturation target in extremely preterm infants. N Engl J Med 2011;364(17):1681; with permission. Copyright © 2011, Massachusetts Medical Society.)

When all 3631 infants were included in the analysis, the infants randomized to Spo_2 of 91% to 95% had greater survival to 36 weeks. Mortality was 17.3% with the low target and 14.4% with the higher target ($P = .015$). Considering only the 1055 infants treated with the revised oximeters, there was a larger survival advantage to targeting higher Spo_2. Mortality was 21.8% in infants targeted to lower Spo_2 versus 13.3% in infants targeted to higher Spo_2 (relative risk for survival with higher Spo_2 1.65, 99.73% CI 1.09–2.49, $P<.001$). A test of interaction was highly significant, suggesting that the treatment effects observed with the original and revised oximeter calibration algorithms were significantly different ($P = .006$). In view of the substantial survival advantage associated with targeting higher Spo_2, recruitment to the BOOST II trials in the United Kingdom and Australia was halted. The other NeoPROM trials had already completed recruitment. It was concluded that, pending the results of longer term follow-up, it was prudent not to target Spo_2 of 85% to 89% in preterm infants.

Considering only the results obtained before the revision of the oximeter calibration algorithm, in the 2576 infants recruited to the 3 BOOST trials and the SUPPORT trial, mortality was not different between Spo_2 treatment groups. The revision of the oximeter calibration algorithm eliminated an unphysiologic artifact and the results obtained after this revision are likely to be more generalizable to clinical practice than the earlier results. If the oximeters had not been revised, it is possible that an incorrect conclusion that targeting Spo_2 less than 90% had no effect on mortality would have been reached, potentially repeating the errors from earlier in the oxygen story.

NEOPROM TRIALS: SUPPORT TRIAL OUTCOMES AT 18 TO 22 MONTHS

The SUPPORT trial has recently published follow-up data to 18 to 22 months.[33] The primary composite outcome for the longer term analysis was death before assessment at 18 to 22 months or neurodevelopmental impairment at 18 to 22 months corrected age.[33] There was no significant difference between the higher-oxygen-saturation group and the lower-oxygen-saturation group for the primary composite outcome. However, mortality was higher in the lower-oxygen-saturation group (22.1% vs 18.2%, relative risk for lower saturation 1.25, 95% CI 1.00–1.55, $P = .046$).

Five of 479 (1.0%) infants in the lower-oxygen-saturation group and 6/511 (1.2%) infants in the higher-oxygen-saturation group were bilaterally blind (visual acuity <20/200) at 18 to 22 months' follow-up ($P = .86$). Thus, although the rates of acute, severe ROP were higher in the higher-oxygen-saturation group,[31] at 18 to 22 months' follow-up there were no differences between the two oxygen-saturation groups in the rates of blindness.[33]

Additional ophthalmic outcomes were available from the neurodevelopment assessments. Strabismus was found in 9.6% of infants in the lower-oxygen-saturation group and in 8.0% of infants in the higher-oxygen-saturation group ($P = .38$). These rates are similar to those reported in low-risk prethreshold cases in the Early Treatment of Retinopathy of Prematurity (ETROP) study, in which 9.6% of infants had strabismus during the first year of life.[34] Corrective lenses for both eyes were needed by 4.5% of infants in the lower-oxygen-saturation group and 4.1% of infants in the higher-oxygen-saturation group. Previous ophthalmic studies have shown a relationship between the severity of acute ROP and the subsequent development of myopia, and have shown progression of myopia over time.[35]

The results of the SUPPORT trial and the preliminary data from the three BOOST II trials show that targeting lower Spo_2 is associated with a significantly higher mortality risk. There is a need to await the follow-up data from all of the trials because, although there was no difference between groups in later neurodevelopmental impairment in the SUPPORT trial, it is possible that this could still be observed in the other trials in infants treated with the revised oximeters.

Higher levels of oxygen saturation during the first few weeks of life result in an increased rate of severe ROP requiring treatment. However, effective treatment of most cases of severe ROP is now available,[36] so the clinical priority is survival. A small number of treatment failures continue to occur, as has been shown in previous ophthalmic treatment trials,[36] and in the SUPPORT study.[33]

FURTHER WORK

The full results of the studies in the NeoPROM collaboration are awaited. Further trials will be necessary. It is unlikely that the same Po_2 or saturation is ideal throughout gestation. It is unlikely that these trials have chanced on the approach that optimizes survival. It is important to recognize that, when oxygen was targeted to measurements of Po_2, the range in common use was 50 to 80 mm Hg. The historical switch to using Spo_2 monitoring that occurred with little supporting evidence was associated with a substantial shift downwards in Po_2. Spo_2 values less than 90% commonly permit Po_2 less than 40 mm Hg (**Fig. 4**).[15,37] A meticulous analysis of the oxygenation patterns over time that are associated with different adverse outcomes is required to inform the way forward. Any new interventions that affect oxygenation, such as closed-loop oxygen control systems should be evaluated carefully. The hope expressed in the 1950s

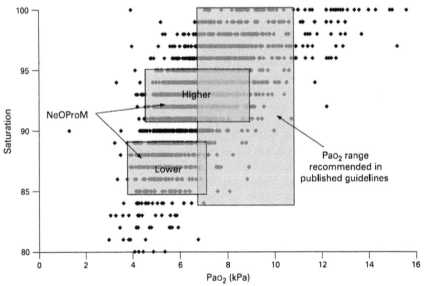

Fig. 4. Spo_2 plotted against Pao_2 from 2076 arterial blood gas specimens taken from oxygen-dependent preterm infants. At each Spo_2 the 95% CIs of Pao_2 for a given Spo_2 could be calculated. The smaller shaded boxes labeled higher and lower represent estimates of the likely 95% CI of Pao_2 for the Spo_2 values in the lower and higher Spo_2 groups in the Neo-PROM trials. The larger shaded box shows the Pao_2 range 50 to 80 mm Hg as recommended in historical guidelines. (*From* Quine D, Stenson BJ. Arterial oxygen tension (Pao_2) values in infants <29 weeks of gestation at currently targeted saturations. Arch Dis Child Fetal Neonatal Ed 2009;95:F52(37), with permission; and *Data from* Myers TR, American Association for Respiratory C. AARC Clinical Practice Guideline: selection of an oxygen delivery device for neonatal and pediatric patients–2002 revision & update. Respir Care 2002;47(6):707–16.)

that ROP might be eliminated by oxygen restriction[8] must now be abandoned. Other approaches to reducing the incidence of severe ROP are needed.

REFERENCES

1. Terry TL. Fibroblastic overgrowth of persistent tunica vasculosa lentis in infants born prematurely: II. Report of cases-clinical aspects. Trans Am Ophthalmol Soc 1942;40:262–84.
2. Campbell K. Intensive oxygen therapy as a possible cause of retrolental fibroplasia; a clinical approach. Med J Aust 1951;2(2):48–50.
3. Patz A, Hoeck LE, De La Cruz E. Studies on the effect of high oxygen administration in retrolental fibroplasia. I. Nursery observations. Am J Ophthalmol 1952; 35(9):1248–53.
4. Ashton N. Animal experiments in retrolental fibroplasia. Trans Am Acad Ophthalmol Otolaryngol 1954;58(1):51–3 [discussion: 53–4].
5. Ashton N. Retrolental fibroplasia. Am J Ophthalmol 1955;39(4 Pt 2):153–9.
6. Askie LM, Henderson-Smart DJ, Ko H. Restricted versus liberal oxygen exposure for preventing morbidity and mortality in preterm or low birth weight infants [meta-analysis review]. Cochrane Database Syst Rev 2009;(1):CD001077.
7. Kinsey VE. Retrolental fibroplasia; cooperative study of retrolental fibroplasia and the use of oxygen. AMA Arch Ophthalmol 1956;56(4):481–543.
8. Guy LP, Lanman JT, Dancis J. The possibility of total elimination of retrolental fibroplasia by oxygen restriction. Pediatrics 1956;17(2):247–9.
9. Cross KW. Cost of preventing retrolental fibroplasia? Lancet 1973;2(7835):954–6.
10. Kinsey VE, Arnold HJ, Kalina RE, et al. Pao$_2$ levels and retrolental fibroplasia: a report of the cooperative study. Pediatrics 1977;60(5):655–68.
11. Yu VY, Hookham DM, Nave JR. Retrolental fibroplasia–controlled study of 4 years' experience in a neonatal intensive care unit. Arch Dis Child 1982;57(4):247–52.
12. Bancalari E, Flynn J, Goldberg RN, et al. Influence of transcutaneous oxygen monitoring on the incidence of retinopathy of prematurity. Pediatrics 1987;79(5):663–9.
13. Flynn JT, Bancalari E, Snyder ES, et al. A cohort study of transcutaneous oxygen tension and the incidence and severity of retinopathy of prematurity. Trans Am Ophthalmol Soc 1991;89:77–92 [discussion: 92–5].
14. Myers TR, American Association for Respir Care. AARC Clinical Practice Guideline: selection of an oxygen delivery device for neonatal and pediatric patients–2002 revision & update. Respir Care 2002;47(6):707–16.
15. Quine D, Stenson BJ. Does the monitoring method influence stability of oxygenation in preterm infants? A randomised crossover study of saturation versus transcutaneous monitoring. Arch Dis Child Fetal Neonatal Ed 2008;93(5):F347–50.
16. Cunningham S, Fleck BW, Elton RA, et al. Transcutaneous oxygen levels in retinopathy of prematurity. Lancet 1995;346(8988):1464–5.
17. Tin W, Milligan DW, Pennefather P, et al. Pulse oximetry, severe retinopathy, and outcome at one year in babies of less than 28 weeks gestation. Arch Dis Child Fetal Neonatal Ed 2001;84(2):F106–10.
18. Anderson CG, Benitz WE, Madan A. Retinopathy of prematurity and pulse oximetry: a national survey of recent practices. J Perinatol 2004;24(3):164–8.
19. Chan-Ling T, Gock B, Stone J. The effect of oxygen on vasoformative cell division. Evidence that 'physiological hypoxia' is the stimulus for normal retinal vasculogenesis. Invest Ophthalmol Vis Sci 1995;36(7):1201–14.
20. Fleck BW, McIntosh N. Pathogenesis of retinopathy of prematurity and possible preventive strategies [review]. Early Hum Dev 2008;84(2):83–8.

21. Hellstrom A, Engstrom E, Hard AL, et al. Postnatal serum insulin-like growth factor I deficiency is associated with retinopathy of prematurity and other complications of premature birth. Pediatrics 2003;112(5):1016–20.
22. Hellstrom A, Perruzzi C, Ju M, et al. Low IGF-I suppresses VEGF-survival signaling in retinal endothelial cells: direct correlation with clinical retinopathy of prematurity. Proc Natl Acad Sci U S A 2001;98(10):5804–8.
23. Supplemental Therapeutic Oxygen for Prethreshold Retinopathy Of Prematurity (STOP-ROP), a randomized, controlled trial. I: primary outcomes. Pediatrics 2000;105(2):295–310.
24. Chow LC, Wright KW, Sola A, Group COAS. Can changes in clinical practice decrease the incidence of severe retinopathy of prematurity in very low birth weight infants? Pediatrics 2003;111(2):339–45.
25. Askie LM, Henderson-Smart DJ, Irwig L, et al. Oxygen-saturation targets and outcomes in extremely preterm infants. N Engl J Med 2003;349(10):959–67.
26. Askie LM, Brocklehurst P, Darlow BA, et al. NeOProM: neonatal oxygenation prospective meta-analysis collaboration study protocol. BMC Pediatr 2011;11:6.
27. Newburger JW, Silbert AR, Buckley LP, et al. Cognitive function and age at repair of transposition of the great arteries in children. N Engl J Med 1984;310(23): 1495–9.
28. Skinner JR, Hunter S, Poets CF, et al. Haemodynamic effects of altering arterial oxygen saturation in preterm infants with respiratory failure. Arch Dis Child Fetal Neonatal Ed 1999;80(2):F81–7.
29. Subhedar NV, Shaw NJ. Changes in pulmonary arterial pressure in preterm infants with chronic lung disease. Arch Dis Child Fetal Neonatal Ed 2000;82(3): F243–7.
30. Johnston ED, Boyle B, Juszczak E, et al. Oxygen targeting in preterm infants using the Masimo SET Radical pulse oximeter. Arch Dis Child Fetal Neonatal Ed 2011;96(6):F429–33.
31. SUPPORT Study Group of the Eunice Kennedy Shriver NICHD Neonatal Research Network, Carlo WA, Finer NN, Walsh MC, et al. Target ranges of oxygen saturation in extremely preterm infants. N Engl J Med 2010;362(21):1959–69.
32. Stenson B, Brocklehurst P, Tarnow-Mordi W, et al. Increased 36-week survival with high oxygen saturation target in extremely preterm infants. N Engl J Med 2011; 364(17):1680–2.
33. Vaucher YE, Peralta-Carcelen M, Finer NN, et al. Neurodevelopmental outcomes in the early CPAP and pulse oximetry trial. N Engl J Med 2012;367(26):2495–504.
34. VanderVeen DK, Coats DK, Dobson V, et al. Prevalence and course of strabismus in the first year of life for infants with prethreshold retinopathy of prematurity: findings from the Early Treatment for Retinopathy of Prematurity study. Arch Ophthalmol 2006;124(6):766–73.
35. Quinn GE, Dobson V, Davitt BV, et al. Progression of myopia and high myopia in the early treatment for retinopathy of prematurity study: findings to 3 years of age. Ophthalmology 2008;115(6):1058–1064.e1.
36. Early Treatment For Retinopathy Of Prematurity Cooperative Group. Revised indications for the treatment of retinopathy of prematurity: results of the early treatment for retinopathy of prematurity randomized trial. Arch Ophthalmol 2003; 121(12):1684–94.
37. Quine D, Stenson BJ. Arterial oxygen tension (Pao_2) values in infants <29 weeks of gestation at currently targeted saturations. Arch Dis Child Fetal Neonatal Ed 2009;94(1):F51–3.

The Challenge of Screening for Retinopathy of Prematurity

Clare M. Wilson, MRCOphth, PhD[a],*, Anna L. Ells, MD, FRCS(C)[b],
Alistair R. Fielder, FRCP, FRCS, FRCOphth[c]

KEYWORDS

- Retinopathy of prematurity screening
- Screening guidelines for retinopathy of prematurity • Telemedicine
- Retinopathy of prematurity

KEY POINTS

- A comprehensive guideline framework for retinopathy of prematurity (ROP) screening is presented, in the hope that the approach is applicable to all countries, though requiring country-specific amendments.
- Telemedicine offers a solution to many of the current geographic and resource problems currently preventing a comprehensive ROP screening program throughout the world.
- Future add-ons to telemedicine such as weight-gain algorithms twinned with quantified vessel analysis could provide automated screening, and this may be a cost-effective solution to the current screening challenge of manpower.

INTRODUCTION

Screening for retinopathy of prematurity (ROP) presents many interesting conundrums. One fundamental consideration deserving reflection is whether clinicians are performing a true screening service when examining for ROP in neonates at risk. Screening implies that a disease is tested for using a simple, safe, noninvasive, and valid test to identify a gold-standard diagnosis. Does the lack of a gold-standard diagnosis in ROP bring into question whether ROP screening should take place, or whether the process should more correctly be named a "case detection initiative?"[1]

Aside from this somewhat cerebral and skeptical query of nomenclature, there are many more practical challenges secondary to the diversity of disease. Broadly these issues fall into 2 categories: (1) which babies should be screened, and (2) how the

[a] Department of Visual Neuroscience, UCL Institute of Ophthalmology, 11–43 Bath Street, London EC1V 9EL, UK; [b] Department of Ophthalmology, University of Calgary, 2500 University Dr NW, Calgary, AB T2N 1N4, Canada; [c] Department of Optometry and Visual Science, City University, Northampton Square, London EC1V 0HB, UK
* Corresponding author.
E-mail address: clare.wilson@ucl.ac.uk

Clin Perinatol 40 (2013) 241–259
http://dx.doi.org/10.1016/j.clp.2013.02.003   perinatology.theclinics.com

babies should be screened. The diversity of ROP presentation is exemplified in its geographic distribution, with variations in the infants at risk and altered temporal development of disease in different locations. The risk of ROP is ubiquitous among the premature neonatal population; the only countries largely exempt are those unable to provide survival care for their preterm infants. The neonatal care needs to be understood for each country. In high-income countries in the late 1950s, the first epidemic of ROP occurred in relatively high birth weight (BW) and gestational age (GA) babies as they were treated with high oxygen concentrations within the neonatal intensive care units (NICUs), as the dangers of oxygen to the eye were not realized. Unfortunately, today in many low-income and middle-income countries supplemental oxygen levels are not monitored, leading to the manifestation of ROP in similarly high GA, high BW infants in these countries, as in the first epidemic.[2]

Further ROP screening challenges worth discussion and in need of resolution include ensuring that the manpower needed to perform the ROP examinations is available, and validating nonclinician lead screening, for example, using remote image transfer further assisted by arguable levels of computerized automation.

Having painted a bleak picture of challenges and obstacles, it should be emphasized that much effort in designing programs to effectively detect infants needing treatment for ROP has been overwhelmingly successful in developed nations.

In this article the authors suggest a framework for ROP "screening" that could be a template for all countries, and postulate some future developments that may standardize and facilitate the screening of ROP within our daily practice.

SCREENING GUIDELINES

That treatment improved the outcome for severe ROP was first reported in 1988,[3] and this made ROP screening and treatment a priority. In the United Kingdom, for instance, in the early 1980s fewer than 10 ophthalmologists were involved in ROP screening, but by 1995, 183 ophthalmologists screened for ROP in 96% of units in the United Kingdom caring for preterm infants.[4] ROP screening is included in the Action Plan 2006-2011 in *Vision 2020 The Right to Sight Global Initiative for the Elimination of Avoidable Blindness*,[5] with the overall aim of providing services to treat children with ROP and with 3 specific strategies: first, "examine premature infants at risk of ROP, treat those with severe disease and promote oxygen monitoring." Second, "ensure availability of ophthalmologists experienced in indirect ophthalmoscopy to identify premature infants in intensive neonatal care who require treatment for ROP." Third, "ensure that infants at risk have fundus examinations starting at 4 to 6 weeks after birth and that infants with severe disease are treated immediately by laser or cryotherapy."[5]

Many countries have devised ROP screening programs and guidelines,[6] a selection of which are listed in **Table 1**. This article does not discuss these in detail, focusing instead on the 2 fundamental principles of screening: which babies, and when, to screen. To this end selected guidelines are cited only to highlight specific issues, and an attempt is made to determine whether there is a global one-fit-all guideline and, if not, whether deviations exist in detail or concept. Here, the terms low-, middle-, and high-income countries are used, but the authors emphasize that this does not always precisely equate to the quality of care in every NICU in a particular country. In high-income countries such as the United States and United Kingdom, the standard of neonatal care is high and although there will be variations, these will probably be relatively minor in comparison with certain other countries such as India, South Africa, and Brazil where the standard of care may vary widely between

Table 1
A selection of screening criteria for ROP from around the globe

Country	Gestational Age (wk) and Body Weight (g)	Notes
Argentina[79]	≤32 wk and/or 1500 g	Include also 1500–2000 g with unstable clinical course, predisposing factors or prolonged oxygen therapy
Brazil[20]	≤32 wk and/or ≤1500 g	Include also larger and more mature babies with illnesses and other risk factors, eg, sepsis, respiratory problems, multiple births
Canada[11]	<31 wk and <1251 g	Include also babies 1251–2000 g if at high risk owing to complex clinical course
Chile[80]	<33 wk and <1500 g	Include also babies between 1500 and 2000 g with unstable clinical course, predisposing risk factor, or prolonged oxygen therapy
Sweden[10]	<31 wk	Include also larger babies severely ill
India[21]	<34 wk and/or <1750 g	Include also babies 34–36 wk or 1750–2000 g if there are risk factors
UK[8]	<31 wk or <1251 g; 1 criterion to be met	Must be screened. No additional sickness criteria
UK[8]	31 to <32 wk or 1251–1501 g; 1 criterion to be met	Should be screened
USA[9]	≤30 wk or <1500 g	Include also "selected" 1500–2000 g or >30 wk if unstable clinical course with cardiorespiratory support and at high risk

individual NICUs, even in one city, from the highest standard in well-resourced units to those with sparse resources in which unblended oxygen is administered. For example, Zin and colleagues[7] mention that in Rio de Janeiro the better NICUs were able to use narrower guidelines than those used other units in the same city.

To set the scene for this section, the descriptors of ROP are briefly described in **Box 1** (**Fig. 1** shows the blood vessels extending from the optic disc) and the indications for treatment are listed in **Box 2**. **Fig. 2** shows classic stage 3 ROP, and **Fig. 3** illustrates aggressive posterior ROP (AP-ROP) with florid vessel congestion and tortuosity of plus disease.

Purpose of ROP Screening

To identify ROP that may require treatment.

Which Babies Need to be Screened?

The first and perhaps major challenge to be faced in ROP screening is determining which babies need to be screened (see **Box 2**). In contrast to many screening activities whereby the individuals at risk have to be identified across the community, all preterm babies at risk for ROP are resident at some time in the NICU and are readily accessible for examination; therefore, omitting to screen the baby who subsequently becomes visually disabled is particularly difficult for the family to understand.

Box 1
Describing ROP

ROP is described by 4 major parameters according to the International Classification of ROP first devised in 1984[76] and then revised in 2005[77,78]

i. Severity by Stage (1–5)

Stages 1 and 2: seen as a demarcation line and ridge, respectively, at the junction of vascularized and avascular retina. Termed mild because, provided they do not progress, they resolve without serious sequelae.

Stage 3: a ridge with extraretinal fibrovascular proliferation. ROP stages 3 to 5 are referred to as being severe because even if treatment is not required, there is a significant risk of ophthalmic sequelae.

Stages 4 and 5: represent partial and total retinal detachment, respectively, and result in severe permanent visual impairment.

Aggressive posterior ROP (AP-ROP): in addition to the stages described above, a new ROP type was described in 2005.[77] The features of AP-ROP are: location in *either* Zone I or posterior Zone II, dilatation and tortuosity of posterior pole retinal vessels out of all proportion to the peripheral retinopathy, which is so subtle and featureless that it can easily be overlooked.

- The term classic ROP is frequently used to denote ROP progressing through the stages and to distinguish this type from AP-ROP.

ii. ROP Extent

Recorded in "clock hours" of the retinal circumference.

iii. Location of ROP Along the Anteroposterior Meridian

Retinal blood vessels grow from Zone I to Zone III, with a high propensity for Zone I ROP to become sight-threatening, whereas for Zone III this is minimal.

iv. Preplus and Plus Disease

A powerful indicator of the activity of the ROP process. The signs of plus disease in order of presentation and increasing severity are: engorgement and tortuosity of the retinal blood vessels near the optic disc, engorgement of the blood vessels of the iris, failure of the pupil to dilate with eye drops (pupil rigidity), and finally, vitreous haze (see **Fig. 1**).

High-income countries

In high-income countries, with a relatively uniform high level of neonatal care, there have been 2 approaches to devising inclusion criteria-based on GA and BW alone, and GA and BW combined with sickness criteria.

GA and BW alone In preparation for the 2008 United Kingdom guideline,[8] data from 10,481 babies, of whom 643 developed sight-threatening ROP, were analyzed. All babies fell within the existing inclusion criteria used in the 1990 and 1995 guidelines of less than 32 weeks GA and/or 1500 g or greater BW, but without a sickness criterion. Had the GA criterion been reduced by 1 week or the BW by 250 g, respectively, 9 babies requiring treatment would have been missed (1 published and 8 known to the Guideline Committee). Accordingly, the criteria were not changed substantially (see **Table 1**) but a lower level of recommendation, "should" be screened, was made for babies between 31 and 32 weeks GA and 1251 to 1501 g BW.

GA and BW combined with sickness criteria This approach, which is used in the United States,[9] Sweden,[10] and Canada,[11] permits lower GA and BW criteria than those of the United Kingdom but requires knowledge of the additional risk factors that pose a risk for ROP. As yet there are very few data on the specificity of illness

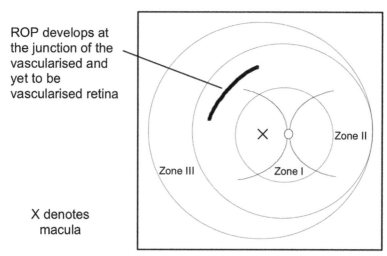

ROP develops at
the junction of the
vascularised and
yet to be
vascularised retina

X denotes
macula

Fig. 1. Blood vessels extend from the optic disc (*central small circle*), first through retinal Zone I, toward Zone III. Acute ROP develops at the growing tips of the blood vessels.

factors that are risk factors for ROP.[12] In the SWEDROP study, which set the current criteria, 2 babies had stage 3 ROP of 32 weeks GA, and the investigators suggest a "strong recommendation to neonatologists to refer also older (ie, higher GA and heavier BW) if they are generally ill or have several comorbidities."[10] It is pertinent to note that in high-income countries with excellent neonatal care, inappropriately excessive oxygen administration is rare (not denying the importance of oxygen in ROP pathogenesis) and the additional risk factors are likely to be sepsis, transfusions, general sickness, prolonged cardiorespiratory support, and so forth, which are most probably nonspecific indicators of illness rather than specific contributors to the ROP process itself, although the authors recognize this is open to debate.

The current inclusion criteria in high-income countries are generally satisfactory. Almost all ROP requiring treatment affects babies of less than 31 weeks GA, or less than 1250 g BW, but it does occasionally occur in larger and more mature babies.[8,12,13] More data are required to determine whether the safest, most effective, and efficient method to include the outliers is by raising the GA and BW bar and ignoring a sickness score, or by setting it at a lower level and combining GA and BW with a "sickness" criterion that will robustly identify the larger baby.

Low-income and middle-income countries
In these countries, with variations in the standard of neonatal care, larger and more mature babies are at risk of developing sight-threatening ROP[1,14–17] in comparison with those in high-income countries. Recent publications from India[17–19] serve to illustrate the issue, with babies of less than 36 weeks GA and greater than 2500 g BW requiring treatment. It is clear that basing inclusion criteria on GA and BW alone under these circumstances would be inappropriate, as many babies would be unnecessarily screened and the demand on ophthalmic services for screening simply could not be met. It should be noted that in some circumstances GA is unknown. As indicated in **Table 1**, the GA and BW inclusion criteria are wider in those middle-income countries that have guidelines such as Brazil[20] and India,[21] but even so, additional sickness criteria are required to identify the larger and more mature babies falling outwith these

Box 2
Indications for ROP treatment

- As a result of the CRYO-ROP study,[3] the criterion for treatment was "Threshold" ROP, defined as the stage at which the risk of blindness if untreated is estimated to be 50%.

- Threshold ROP has a specific meaning in the ROP world, and was the indication for treatment between 1988 and late 2003 when it was superseded by the revised recommendations for treatment proposed by the Early Treatment for Retinopathy of Prematurity Cooperative Group,[77] referred to as Prethreshold but including Threshold as defined above.

These 2 indications for treatment are:

Threshold ROP (CRYO-ROP), 1988 to December 2003:

    At least 5 continuous or 8 cumulative clock hours of stage 3 ROP

    In Zones I or II, and in the presence of plus disease

ETROP (Early Treatment for Retinopathy of Prematurity) Recommendations for Treatment, December 2003 onwards:

Type I ROP

    Zone I, any stage of ROP with plus disease and stage 3 without plus disease

    Zone II, stage 2 or 3 with plus disease

Type II ROP

    Zone I, stage 1 or 2 ROP without plus disease

    Zone II, stage 3 ROP without plus disease

The ETROP recommendation was that Type I eyes should be treated as soon as possible ("promptly"). Thus, AP-ROP should be treated within 24 to 48 hours, whereas other forms of ROP requiring treatment but which are not AP-ROP should be treated within 48 to 72 hours (United Kingdom guideline)

- Type II eyes should be watched and treated if there is progression to Type I ROP.

- ROP may be treated by either cryotherapy or laser, but over the past decade or so laser has been used almost exclusively.

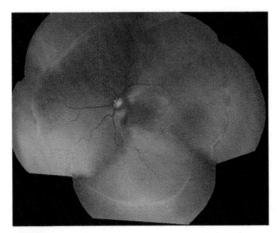

Fig. 2. Classic stage 3 ROP.

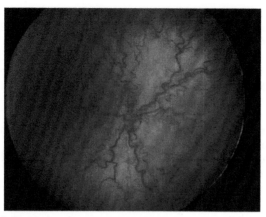

Fig. 3. AP-ROP with florid plus disease.

criteria. Inappropriate excessive oxygen administration, sometimes unblended, has long been suspected to be a factor, although, unsurprisingly, robust clinical data are usually missing. Shah and colleagues[18] recently reported a high incidence of AP-ROP in babies of less than 35 weeks GA who had received unblended oxygen and that, following crude oxygen blending, this incidence fell dramatically, thus conclusively proving that in these babies at least, oxygen was the dominant risk factor for ROP.

Inclusion criteria: final comments
Whereas neonatal care in high-income countries is relatively uniformly excellent (in this context), in middle- and low-income countries care may range from excellent to low between NICUs, even in one city; thus, as stated earlier, the income of the country does not describe the full picture of individual units. Furthermore, neonatal management is continually changing, so reevaluation of inclusion criteria will be necessary from time to time. Local audit is an essential component but, although the results can be used to broaden criteria, making them narrower, on what may be a relatively small evidence base, should be undertaken with caution.

When to Screen?

ROP natural history
An effective and efficient screening program requires understanding of the natural history of ROP, and this has been studied in population-based[22–24] and treatment studies.[25–27] Findings have been very consistent over a 20-year period, showing that the onset and progression of ROP are governed predominantly by postmenstrual age (PMA) and not postnatal age, although there is a slight acceleration of the process in the most immature babies.[24] The rate of progress through the stages is approximately 1 stage per 7 to 10 days: thus in ETROP,[27] the median age for stages 1, 2, and 3, and plus disease was 34.1, 35.1, 36.6, and 36.0 weeks PMA, respectively. ROP very rarely requires treatment before 31 weeks PMA and the mean age for treatment of Type I (prethreshold) and threshold disease in ETROP[28] was 35.2 weeks PMA (range 30.6–42.1 weeks) and 37.0 weeks PMA (range 31.9–46.6 weeks), essentially identical to previous studies.

So far ROP natural history has only been considered in preterm populations with a high standard of neonatal care whereby the risk of severe disease is confined to babies lighter than 1250 to 1500 g BW. With respect to larger babies, Carden and colleagues[15] reported on 100 preterm babies of less than 1900 g BW and less than 35 weeks GA in Vietnam, who required treatment for threshold ROP at 36.25 weeks PMA (range 31.4–44.3 weeks). From India, Shah and colleagues[18] reported laser treatment to 93 babies (<2250 g BW and <35 weeks GA) at mean age of 37 weeks PMA (range 30–40 weeks), and Jalali and colleagues[19] treated 115 babies with AP-ROP at a mean age of 34.6 weeks PMA (range 31–51 weeks PMA). Thus the information to date confirms that the natural history of ROP is governed by PMA, so that the mean age of babies requiring treatment at threshold ROP is around 37 weeks and at prethreshold around 35 weeks, even in larger babies. It follows that progression through the stages will be compressed in the larger babies, of which there are anecdotal examples and the National Neonatology Foundation of India guideline, which recommends screening by 2 to 3 weeks of age.[21]

When to start screening
Screening should commence before ROP requires treatment. Several ROP guidelines have given a single postnatal age for the commencement of screening examinations, for example, 6 to 7 weeks for the 1995 United Kingdom guideline[29] and 4 to 6 weeks in the Vision 2020 Action Plan.[5] Although this had the merit of simplicity, it did not take into consideration the natural history of ROP and consequently required excessive examinations of the most immature babies, yet would have missed the opportunity for treatment in the largest and most mature baby. Several national guidelines have now followed the approach suggested by Reynolds and colleagues[26] whereby the commencement of screening is tailored to the baby's GA. This guideline is shown in **Table 2** and has been extended beyond 32 weeks for the purpose of this article. It is especially important to examine larger babies earlier.

When screening can be safely terminated
The decision to terminate screening safely is obviously crucial, and should be considered in 2 circumstances.

Table 2
At what age should first screening examination take place?

| | Age at First ROP Screening Examination | |
Gestational Age (wk)	Postnatal Age (wk)	Postmenstrual Age (wk)
22	8	30
23	7	30
24	6	30
25	5	30
26	4	30
27	4	31
28	4	32
29	4	33
30	4	34
31	4	35
32	3	35
33	2	35
34	2	36
35	2	37

The baby without ROP Several guidelines have recommended that screening should be continued until full vascularization is achieved. The authors consider this difficult to achieve and unlikely to be obeyed. It is agreed that once retinal vascularization has reached Zone III, the risk of a serious adverse outcome is minimal. However, the accurate identification of the zone can be difficult and is prone to error. For this reason the United Kingdom guideline recommends screening until the 37th postmenstrual week has been entered.[8] Whether screening needs to be continued for longer in the larger baby is not known.

The baby with ROP Signs of regression on at least 2 examinations.

TOWARD A GLOBAL GUIDELINE

The past 2 decades has seen great advances in our understanding of how ROP behaves. Several national guidelines have been produced, and these have evolved with each iteration. Both undercompliance and overcompliance with guidelines has been reported,[30] and problems with screening are a major source of medicolegal concern.[31] **Table 3** is a highly simplistic attempt to present ROP causation as an equation. As described, with a high standard of neonatal care the major risk factor for ROP is the degree of prematurity and under this circumstance, ROP onset and progression are governed predominantly by PMA with "sickness" and oxygen administration playing relatively minor, albeit important roles. When neonatal care is of a lower standard, especially when unblended oxygen is administered, the equation can be totally swamped by oxygen, causing severe (sometimes AP-ROP) ROP in large babies in good condition. The possibility cannot be ignored that in these circumstances, ROP progresses more rapidly than with a high standard of neonatal care, although the literature to date does not support such a contention.

The Global Guideline

A one-fits-all global guideline is not quite as far-fetched as might be thought. Undoubtedly there will be differences in detail, but the underlying concepts are probably universal. Here the authors make a tentative (emphasis on this word) attempt to consider how a one-fits-all guideline might be devised.

Which babies should be screened

This aspect requires understanding of the babies at risk in each locality, mindful of the dangers of relying on a small database. The approach adopted by several countries seems sensible: to set the GA and BW characteristics that would include all or most of the babies at risk in that location. A local trade-off between effectiveness and efficiency needs to be struck. In addition, the inclusion of a sickness criterion needs to be considered so that any babies at risk but not covered by these criteria are identified. It would appear that where there is high-quality neonatal care, the sickness criteria are indicators of the complications of extreme prematurity and perhaps not all causally related to ROP, whereas where care is of a lower standard and particularly when

Table 3 The ROP equation					
Standard of Neonatal Care	Immaturity	"Sickness"	Oxygen Administration	=	ROP
High	+++++	+(+)	++		
Variable	+++	?	+++++		

unblended oxygen is given, the sickness criterion can be a specific factor in ROP causation.

The timing of ROP screening

The start of screening needs to be timed according to the schedule in **Table 2**. It is most unlikely that this needs amended according to meet local circumstances, but this statement is made with one important caveat: the possibility that very preterm babies receiving unblended oxygen may develop severe ROP rapidly. This likelihood is not supported by the literature to date, but further research is required. In the absence of any ROP, screening can be terminated when the retinal vessels are well into Zone III, which in high-income countries is at least 37 weeks PMA, but might need to continue a week or so longer in larger babies. More data on this point are needed.

To conclude, the principles of ROP screening are common to all communities, but there are differences of detail, especially with respect to the identification of babies who need to be screened. Furthermore, with advances in both our understanding of ROP and neonatal management, fine tuning of guidelines will be required from time to time.

TELEMEDICINE APPROACH TO ROP

Telemedicine refers to the use of information technologies to support health care between participants who are separated from each other, and offers a possible solution to some of the screening challenges in the management of ROP.

Since 2001, research projects using a telemedicine approach to ROP screening have consistently demonstrated the ability to identify infants at risk for severe ROP needing treatment. There are more than 25 peer-reviewed published studies that document the feasibility and accuracy of this approach, and there is not a single case of remote interpretation of ROP images that have not appropriately identified severe disease warranting an on-site diagnostic examination by an ophthalmologist.[32–34]

Furthermore, several telemedicine studies documented identification of severe ROP disease 1 to 2 weeks earlier than the clinical binocular indirect ophthalmoscopy standard.[35,36] Earlier identification of disease leads to earlier treatment of severe ROP, and early treatment results in better visual outcomes.[28,37,38] These studies are consistent with major clinical trials in diabetic retinopathy that document the efficacy of digital imaging with remote evaluation as better than ophthalmologists' examinations in detecting the features of diabetic retinopathy.[39,40] The use of telemedicine to manage infants with ROP offers the potential to address the shortage of physician expertise, standardize and improve the quality of ROP evaluations, and optimize the timing of treatment of premature infants.

Meeting the growing need for efficient, effective, and timely ROP evaluations is international in scope. A recent multicentered, randomized clinical trial (ETROP)[28] studying earlier laser treatment of severe ROP emphasized the need for more frequent examinations to result in accurate and timely diagnosis of treatable disease. However, this has added significantly to the overall burden of ROP evaluations.[27,29] An audit in the United Kingdom in 1997/1998 reported that 55 ROP examinations by an ophthalmologist occurred for every infant who required laser treatment.[30] In Canada and the United States,[41,42] a similar ratio exists between infants examined and infants treated. In Canada, fewer than 100 subspecialists perform more than 12,150 ROP examinations per year.[41]

Advances in imaging techniques have enabled the manufacture of digital cameras specifically for imaging the posterior segment and retina of premature infants. The RetCam digital camera system (Clarity Medical Systems Inc, Pleasanton, CA) is the most commonly used camera for neonatal ophthalmic imaging. The wide-angle lens gives a panoramic view of the retina, and the capture-and-save feature enables photographic documentation of retinal pathology that may become part of the permanent medical record. The additional benefit of the photographic documentation in screening for ROP is its use remotely in telemedicine systems. The RetCam$_3$ has a 130° field of view, with optional 80° and 30° high-magnification interchangeable lenses. It is a charged coupled device camera capturing 640 × 480-pixel, 24-bit, red, green, blue (RGB) bitmap images. It is necessary to dilate the infant's pupils and use topical anesthetic before examination. The eyelids are held open by an eyelid speculum, and the camera probe applanates the corneal surface gently using contact lens gel. Retinal photographic documentation of infants at risk for ROP using the RetCam camera with remote interpretation of digital images has been favorably assessed in many studies of babies, but there has yet to be a large multicenter study published to confirm its ability to produce the same accuracy of ROP disease detection in comparison with the clinical gold standard of indirect ophthalmoscopy.[35,36]

An Ophthalmic Technology Assessment report commissioned by the American Academy of Ophthalmology has evaluated the accuracy of detecting clinically significant ROP using wide-angle digital retinal photography from the literature currently available.[43] It reviewed 7 level I articles and 3 level III articles. Of these 10 articles, 7 reported a high sensitivity and specificity for detecting ROP needing treatment using digital imaging.

Chiang and colleagues[43] also reported on 3 "Real-World ROP Management Programs." These programs have successfully set up ROP telemedicine programs and have published data supporting their validity. The largest published dataset of infants screened for ROP using telemedicine is from Bangalore, India. This telemedicine program, KIDROP (Karnataka Internet Assisted Diagnosis of Retinopathy of Prematurity), has been screening in remote NICUs in rural regions where ROP screening does not exist.[44,45] Trained and certified technicians visit 81 hospitals on a fixed schedule in more than 18 districts of Karnataka state (inhabited by 64 million persons) in 3 defined zones and, using the RetCam Shuttle, image infants who are either resident to that NICU or are referred to the program. Images are stored, analyzed, and uploaded on a secure Tele-ROP platform (i2i Tele-solutions Ltd, Bangalore, India) for the expert to view and report on a smartphone, tablet, or computer, in real time, using a standardized template.[46] Since its inception in 2008, and by the end of 2012, 9058 infants have been cumulatively enrolled for ROP screening, of whom 718 babies (7.9%) have been diagnosed with ETROP grade disease and treated in these remote centers itself, obviating travel for these underprivileged rural babies who would not otherwise have had access to ROP care.[21]

In Germany, Lorenz and colleagues[47] showed 100% detection of suspected treatment-warranted cases. This study comprised prospectively collected data from 1222 infants taken over 6 years at 5 neonatal intensive care units. In California, the Stanford University Network for Diagnosis of ROP has reported 100% sensitivity and 90% specificity at detecting treatment-warranted cases of ROP.[33] A further real-world program in Auckland, New Zealand reported 100% sensitivity at detecting treatment-warranted ROP, and a specificity of 98%.[48] In Montana, Weaver and Murdock[49] have reported that of 137 infants examined by telemedical examinations, 13 infants were transferred for referral-warranted ROP and 9 of them ultimately required laser treatment. No neonate progressed to stage 4 or 5 ROP during the 4.5-year study period.

There is currently an ongoing National Eye Institute multicenter clinical trial due to be completed in May 2015, which compares the accuracy of remote interpretation of digital images of ROP with results from corresponding indirect ophthalmoscopy retinal examinations.[50] The aim is to enroll 2000 babies from 12 centers in the United States and Canada. Babies with a BW of less than 1251 g are included in the study. Digital retinal imaging and clinically indicated indirect ophthalmoscopy are performed on the same day. The RetCam images are taken by certified ROP imagers, and the ophthalmologist performs indirect ophthalmoscopy and records the ROP. Digital ROP images are remotely interpreted via a secure Web-based site by both ophthalmologists and nonphysician graders. The primary outcome measure is the detection of referral-warranted ROP (characteristics of severe disease, possibly requiring treatment) on digital images.

After further multicenter validation of a telemedicine approach for ROP, more information will be required for standardized implementation and evaluation of international telemedicine ROP programs, which will also include the nuances of such care provision that will need to be determined. Some of these issues (eg, the use of trained technicians or nurses to acquire the images) are being addressed in the multicenter trial currently under way.

Once the images have been acquired, the safe storage and transfer of images to the expert ophthalmologist will need to be standardized, along with ROP grading software. The highly intuitive iPhone with customized ROP grading software is currently being evaluated by Vinekar and Ells (personal communication from one of the investigators, A.E., January 2013). The ability to use a smartphone for remote image interpretation would increase access and availability of image interpretation by ROP experts around the world. High-speed Internet access is ideal to enable quick image upload, but the advancing capabilities of 3G and 4G may negate the need for that, which possibly would be of benefit in the rural areas of low-income countries. An alternative approach for the future might be that with advances in retinal vessel analysis, telemedicine might include the transmission of a vessel measurement in addition to the image (see next section).

In summary, a telemedicine approach to ROP would potentially generate a permanent digital image for accurate documentation of ROP (a picture is worth a thousand words), would increase the access of ROP care in both developed and developing countries, and would standardize treatment and, ultimately, prevent or limit vision loss and blindness from ROP around the world.

SEMIAUTOMATED IMAGE ANALYSIS AND ALGORITHMS: THE FUTURE OF ROP SCREENING?

Less than 10% of neonates screened for ROP will require treatment, so the vast majority does not develop ROP, or it is mild and self-limited. This scenario offers 2 options for screening: identifying the eye not at risk of developing sight-threatening ROP, or predicting reliably the eye that is likely to progress. Predictive factors for the likelihood of disease progression can be reliably isolated. Predictive factors for ROP progression studied thus far include postnatal weight gain, levels of serum insulin-like growth factor 1 (IGF-1), and quantifiable vessel changes in the retina. The dichotomous distinction between disease presence and disease absence may be a warranted first step in assessing these babies. There is also growing evidence that genetic factors are linked with disease severity, and in the more distant future, genetic screening may also add to the decision as to which babies are more likely to benefit from eye examinations.

An alternative and complementary approach to identifying either the eye with no/mild or severe ROP is through retinal vessel analysis. Image analysis techniques have progressed rapidly, and over the last decade retinal vessel analysis tools have been developed specifically to assess the vascular changes in the posterior pole associated with plus disease of ROP. Image segmentation isolates areas of interest within an image. There are many different image-segmentation techniques, and these can broadly be divided into ridge-based and region-based techniques. Such techniques have been applied to retinal images by many teams globally to identify blood vessels in images. Locating the tiniest blood vessels in preterm neonates has been challenging for software, but progress is being made, and the accuracy of these systems may consequently equip them to be the most sensitive and specific tools for finding features in adult images. The first reports of semiautomated image analysis techniques for identifying and then quantifying retinal vessels from RetCam images were from Imperial College London, where Retinal Image multiScale Analysis (RISA) had been developed.[51]

RISA vessel segmentation is based on 2 geometric features obtained at different scales by means of Gaussian derivative operators. The geometric features are based on the first and second derivatives of the intensity of the image, maximum gradient, and principal curvature. RISA finds the maxima in scale space, and has an extra constraint on these maxima in that the gradient must be very low, as a starter point for region growing. A multiple-pass region-growing procedure is used, which progressively segments the vessels using the feature information about the 8 neighboring pixels.[51] RISA has been used to quantify arterial tortuosity in ROP,[52] and subsequently showed that in patients with plus disease arteriolar and venous curvature, diameter, and tortuosity index are all increased in comparison with those without plus disease.[53] The rate of change in venous parameters has been correlated with development of plus disease using RISA, with the highest area under the curve reported in venous tortuosity index for weekly rate of change.[54]

A further vessel detection software, ROPtool, has been developed at Duke University, North Carolina. A comparison of ROPtool tortuosity results from 185 RetCam images from preterm babies with 6 pediatric ophthalmologists gradings of plus, preplus, and normal found 97% sensitivity for identifying tortuosity sufficient for plus disease.[55,56] ROPtool has been developed from a program to detect tubular structures in 3-dimensional images such as the intracerebral vasculature from magnetic resonance angiography images.[57] It is based on centerline extraction; when given a start point such as a mouse click, its associated intensity ridge can be found by mapping image intensity to height.[58]

Computer-Aided Image Analysis of the Retina (CAIAR) was developed from RISA to enable quicker image analysis, owing to its more accurate image-segmentation techniques. CAIAR detects vessels in an image using a maximum likelihood model fitting in a scale-space framework. It uses filters sensitive to ridge-like structures at 4 different scales and models that are fitted to the filter outputs to estimate the most likely vessel configuration. Parameters of height, width, and orientation are computed at each point in the image, and an estimated model of Gaussian profile is produced. An isotropic second derivative of Gaussian filter is then used to verify the output, measuring the contrast in a cross section perpendicular to the direction of the vessel and checking that the maximum contrast to the background is in the center of the proposed vessel.[59] CAIAR has been validated using computer-generated vessels with increasing amplitude and frequency (to validate tortuosity readings) and differing widths, and validated clinically using RetCam images of infants undergoing ROP screening and comparing CAIAR width and tortuosity outputs with those of clinician graders.[60] CAIAR has also been validated using smaller field-of-view, higher-resolution images obtained using the Nidek NM200D noncontact camera. Results were compared with disease severity and with results from Vasculo-matic ala Nicola version 1.1 (IVAN), a further vessel-segmentation software that had previously been validated for measurement of vessel width.[61] The stratification of risk of developing progression from preplus to treatment requiring plus in 30 eyes was studied using CAIAR. Of these 30 eyes, 19 regressed and 11 progressed to develop plus disease. The mean width and tortuosity values of the 3 widest or most tortuous vessels, respectively, predicted which eyes would develop to require treatment.[62]

These semiautomated systems can detect plus disease of ROP with accuracy comparable with or even better than that of experts.[63–66] As well as vessel width and tortuosity, other retinal parameters such as vessel branching pattern and arcade angles[67,68] may add strength to automated digital image analysis as a screening tool for ROP.

At present, there are limitations to automated image analysis: while tortuosity can be accurately calculated, width measurements are less robust and all methods are slow. The difficulty for man and machine to distinguish arterioles from venules maybe an unnecessary concern, as the authors have recently shown that the 4 most tortuous vessels in an image, regardless of their vessel type, are correlated well with treated versus untreated eyes.[69] It has been suggested that improved retinal image-segmentation methods, mathematical combinations of individual feature values such as width and tortuosity, and replication of work using larger datasets will rely on multidisciplinary collaborative efforts,[43] but these efforts will surely be worthwhile. There is a need for these programs to be accurate, and a faster, ideally totally automated version producing a quantification of the likelihood of the eye requiring treatment may be ideal.

As described in more detail elsewhere in this ROP issue, WINROP (Weight, IGF-1 levels, Neonatal, ROP) is a surveillance algorithm developed by Lofqvist and colleagues[70] in Sweden. It measures weekly IGF-1 levels and weekly weight from birth until 36 weeks. WINROP correctly identified all babies subsequently requiring laser treatment for proliferative ROP and also all infants with low-risk ROP in a group of 50 preterm infants. A further study of 354 infants in Sweden using only postnatal weight gain showed 100% sensitivity and 84.5% specificity,[71] and this was validated in a United States cohort of 318 infants, again accurately predicting all babies who went on to develop ROP requiring treatment.[72] Binenbaum and colleagues[73] reported that a predictive model based on postnatal weight gain was able to reduce the need for ophthalmoscopic screening.

There is growing evidence that genetic susceptibility plays a role in development of severe ROP. Three genes encoding for the Wnt and Norrin signaling pathways have been described to cause familial exudative vitreoretinopathy (FEVR), and 2 of these have been identified in infants developing ROP: the NDP gene (X-lined FEVR) and the FZD4 gene (autosomal dominant FEVR). Ells and colleagues[74] identified 2 novel mutations (Ala370Gly and Lys203Asn) in the FZD4 gene in 2 of 71 infants with severe ROP. This mutation was not found in the 33 infants in the group with mild to no ROP, or in 173 random Caucasian samples. Mutation in the NDP gene has been calculated to account for 3% of cases of severe ROP.[75]

Image analysis is likely to be a feasible cotside test in the foreseeable future if completely automated and rapid. Attempts to develop CAIAR into an automated program, generating a value of likelihood for progression to treatment requiring disease, is currently under development.[63] Weight gain and image analysis are complementary methods that may facilitate the development of a nonphysician screening program in which the 90% or so infants, who either will never develop ROP or in whom it is mild and self-limiting, can be identified. Only those infants close to developing sight-threatening ROP will then be required to be examined by an ophthalmologist. This method could be a timely and cost-effective way of providing screening in low- and middle-income countries where access is low, and in high-income countries where screening can consume inappropriate amounts of health resources, leading to reluctance to perform this activity in certain areas.

REFERENCES

1. Gilbert C. Retinopathy of prematurity: a global perspective of the epidemics: population of babies at risk and implications for control. Early Hum Dev 2008; 84:77–82.
2. Shah PK, Narendran V, Kalpana N, et al. Severe retinopathy of prematurity in big babies in India: history repeating itself? Indian J Pediatr 2009;76(8):801–4.
3. Cryotherapy for Retinopathy of Prematurity Cooperative Group. Multicentre trial of cryotherapy for retinopathy of prematurity: preliminary results. Arch Ophthalmol 1988;106:471–9.
4. Haines L, Fielder AR, Scrivener R, et al. Retinopathy of prematurity in the UK I: the organisation of services for screening and treatment. Eye (Lond) 2002;16: 33–8.
5. Vision 2020: the Right to Sight. Action plan 2006-2011; IAPB, Vision 2020, WHO. Available at: www.who.int/blindness/Vision2020_report. Accessed January 1, 2013.
6. Ells A, Hicks M, Fielden M, et al. Severe retinopathy of prematurity: longitudinal observation of disease and screening implications. Eye (Lond) 2005;19:138–44.
7. Zin AA, Moreira ME, Bunce C, et al. Retinopathy of prematurity in 7 neonatal units in Rio de Janeiro: screening criteria and workload implications. Pediatrics 2010;126:e410–7.
8. Wilkinson AR, Haines L, Head K, et al. UK retinopathy of prematurity guideline. Early Hum Dev 2008;84:71–4 Guideline in full available at: www.rcpch.ac.uk www.rcophth.ac.uk. Accessed January 1, 2013.
9. American Academy of Pediatrics Section on Ophthalmology, American Academy of Ophthalmology, American Association for Pediatric Ophthalmology and Strabismus, American Association of Certified Orthoptists. Screening examination of premature infants for retinopathy of prematurity. Pediatrics 2013;131: 189–95.
10. Holmström GE, Hellström A, Jakobsson PG, et al. Swedish National Register for Retinopathy of Prematurity (SWEDROP) and the Evaluation of Screening in Sweden. Arch Ophthalmol 2012;130:1418–24.
11. Jefferies AL. Canadian paediatric society, fetus and newborn committee. Paediatr Child Health 2010;15:670.
12. Yanovitch TL, Siatkowski RM, McCaffree M, et al. Retinopathy of prematurity in infants with birth weight > or = 1250 grams—incidence, severity, and screening guideline cost-analysis. J AAPOS 2006;10:128–34.
13. Hutchinson AK, O'Neil JW, Morgan EN, et al. Retinopathy of prematurity in infants with birth weights greater than 1250 grams. J AAPOS 2003;7:190–4.
14. Gilbert C, Fielder A, Gordillo L, et al, International NO-ROP Group. Characteristics of infants with severe retinopathy of prematurity in countries with low, moderate, and high levels of development: implications for screening programs. Pediatrics 2005;115:e518–25.
15. Carden SM, Luu LN, Nguyen TX, et al. Retinopathy of prematurity: postmenstrual age at threshold in a transitional economy is similar to that in developed countries. Clin Experiment Ophthalmol 2008;36:159–61.
16. Chen Y, Li X. Characteristics of severe retinopathy patients in China: a repeat of the first epidemic? Br J Ophthalmol 2006;90:268–71.

17. Vinekar A, Dogra MR, Sangtam T, et al. Retinopathy of prematurity in Asian Indian babies weighing greater than 1250 grams at birth: ten year data from a tertiary care center in a developing country. Indian J Ophthalmol 2007;55:331–6.

18. Shah PK, Narendran V, Kalpana N. Aggressive posterior retinopathy of prematurity in large preterm babies in South India. Arch Dis Child Fetal Neonatal Ed 2012;97:F371–5.

19. Jalali S, Kesarwani S, Hussain A. Outcomes of a protocol-based management for zone I retinopathy of prematurity: the Indian twin cities screening program report number 2. Am J Ophthalmol 2011;151:719–24.

20. Zin A, Florêncio T, Fortes Filho JB, et al, Brazilian Society of Pediatrics, Brazilian Council of Ophthalmology and Brazilian Society of Pediatric Ophthalmology. Brazilian guidelines proposal for screening and treatment of retinopathy of prematurity (ROP). Arq Bras Oftalmol 2007;70:875–83 [in Portuguese].

21. Pejaver RK, Vinekar A, Bilagi A. National Neonatology Foundation's evidence based clinical practice guidelines 2010. Retinopathy prematurity (NNF India, Guidelines). Barwala (Haryana, India): Chandika Press Pvt Ltd; 2010. p. 253–62.

22. Fielder AR, Shaw DE, Robinson J, et al. Natural history of retinopathy of prematurity: a prospective study. Eye 1992;6:233–42.

23. Holmström G, el Azazi M, Jacobson L, et al. A population based, prospective study of the development of ROP in prematurely born children in the Stockholm area of Sweden. Br J Ophthalmol 1993;77:417–23.

24. Austeng D, Källen KB, Hellström A, et al. Natural history of retinopathy of prematurity in infants born before 27 weeks' gestation in Sweden. Arch Ophthalmol 2010;128:1289–94.

25. Palmer EA, Flynn JT, Hardy RJ, et al. The Cryotherapy for Retinopathy of Prematurity Cooperative Group. Incidence and early course of retinopathy of prematurity. Ophthalmology 1991;98:1628–40.

26. Reynolds JD, Dobson V, Quinn GE, et al, on behalf of the CRYO-ROP and LIGHT-ROP Cooperative Groups. Evidence-based screening criteria for retinopathy of prematurity: natural history data from CRYO-ROP and LIGHT-ROP Studies. Arch Ophthalmol 2002;120:1470–6.

27. Good WV, Hardy RJ, Dobson V, et al, Early Treatment for Retinopathy of Prematurity Cooperative Group. The incidence and course of retinopathy of prematurity: findings from the Early Treatment for Retinopathy of Prematurity study. Pediatrics 2005;116:15–23.

28. Good WV, Early Treatment for Retinopathy of Prematurity Cooperative Group. Final results of the Early Treatment for Retinopathy of Prematurity (ETROP) randomized trial. Trans Am Ophthalmol Soc 2004;102:233–50 [discussion: 248–50].

29. Ophthalmologists and British Association of Perinatal Medicine. Early Hum Dev 1996;46:239–58.

30. Fielder AR, Haines L, Scrivener R, et al. Retinopathy of prematurity in the UK II: audit of national guidelines for screening and treatment. Eye (Lond) 2002;16:285–91.

31. Reynolds JD. Malpractice and the quality of care in retinopathy of prematurity (an American Ophthalmological Society thesis). Trans Am Ophthalmol Soc 2007;105:461–80.

32. Chiang MF, Wang L, Busuioc M, et al. Telemedical retinopathy of prematurity diagnosis: accuracy, reliability, and image quality. Arch Ophthalmol 2007;125(11):1531–8.

33. Silva RA, Murakami Y, Jain A, et al. Stanford University Network for Diagnosis of Retinopathy of Prematurity (SUNDROP): 18-month experience with telemedicine screening. Graefes Arch Clin Exp Ophthalmol 2009;247(1):129–36.

34. Wu C, Petersen RA, VanderVeen DK. RetCam imaging for retinopathy of prematurity screening. J AAPOS 2006;10(2):107–11.
35. Ells AL, Holmes JM, Astle WF, et al. Telemedicine approach to screening for severe retinopathy of prematurity: a pilot study. Ophthalmology 2003;110(11):2113–7.
36. Photographic Screening for Retinopathy of Prematurity (Photo-ROP) Cooperative Group. The photographic screening for retinopathy of prematurity study (photo-ROP) primary outcomes. Retina 2008;28(Suppl 3):S47–54.
37. Good WV, Early Treatment for Retinopathy of Prematurity Cooperative Group. The Early Treatment for Retinopathy of Prematurity study: structural findings at age 2 years. Br J Ophthalmol 2006;90(11):1378–82.
38. Hardy RJ, Good WV, Dobson V, et al. The Early Treatment for Retinopathy of Prematurity clinical trial: presentation by subgroups versus analysis within subgroups. Br J Ophthalmol 2006;90(11):1341–2.
39. Fransen SR, Leonard-Martin TC, Feuer WJ, et al. Clinical evaluation of patients with diabetic retinopathy: accuracy of the Inoveon diabetic retinopathy-3DT system. Ophthalmology 2002;109(3):595–601.
40. Lee P. Telemedicine: opportunities and challenges for the remote care of diabetic retinopathy. Arch Ophthalmol 1999;117(12):1639–40.
41. Lee SK, Normand C, McMillan D, et al. Evidence for changing guidelines for routine screening for retinopathy of prematurity. Arch Pediatr Adolesc Med 2001;155(3):387–95.
42. Lee SK, McMillan DD, Ohlsson A, et al. Variations in practice and outcomes in the Canadian NICU network: 1996-1997. Pediatrics 2000;106(5):1070–9.
43. Chiang MF, Melia M, Buffenn AN, et al. Detection of clinically significant retinopathy of prematurity using wide-angle digital retinal photography. Ophthalmology 2012;119:1272–80.
44. Hungi B, Vinekar A, Datti N, et al. Retinopathy of prematurity in a rural neonatal intensive care unit in south India—a prospective study. Indian J Pediatr 2012;79(7):911–5.
45. Vinekar A, Avadhani K, Braganza S, et al. Outcomes of a protocol-based management for zone 1 retinopathy of prematurity: the Indian Twin Cities ROP Screening Program report number 2. Am J Ophthalmol 2011;152(4):712.
46. Vinekar A. IT-enabled innovation to prevent infant blindness in rural India: the KIDROP experience. Journal Indian Business Research 2011;3(2):98–102.
47. Lorenz B, Spasovska K, Elflein H, et al. Wide-field digital imaging based telemedicine for screening for acute retinopathy of prematurity (ROP): six-year results of a multicentre field study. Graefes Arch Clin Exp Ophthalmol 2009;247:1251–62.
48. Dai S, Chow K, Vincent A. Efficacy of wide-field digital retinal imaging for retinopathy of prematurity screening. Clin Experiment Ophthalmol 2011;39:23–9.
49. Weaver DT, Murdock TJ. Telemedicine detection of type 1 ROP in a distant neonatal intensive care unit. J AAPOS 2012;16:229–33.
50. eROP clinical trial. Available at: http://clinicaltrials.gov/ct2/show/NTCO1264276. Accessed January 1, 2013.
51. Martinez-Perez E, Stanton AV, Thorn SA, et al. Retinal vascular tree morphology: a semi-automatic quantification. IEEE Trans Biomed Eng 2002;49(8):912–7.
52. Swanson C, Coker KD, Parker KH, et al. Semiautomated computer analysis of vessel growth in preterm infants without and with retinopathy of prematurity. Br J Ophthalmol 2003;87(12):1474–7.
53. Gelman R, Martinez-Perez ME, Vanderveen DK, et al. Diagnosis of plus disease in retinopathy of prematurity using Retinal Image multiScale Analysis. Invest Ophthalmol Vis Sci 2005;46(12):4734–856.

54. Thyparampil PJ, Park Y, Martinez-Perez ME, et al. Plus disease in retinopathy of prematurity: quantitative analysis of vascular change. Am J Ophthalmol 2010; 150(4):468–75.

55. Wallace DK. Computer-assisted quantification of vascular tortuosity in retinopathy of prematurity (an American Ophthalmological Society thesis). Trans Am Ophthalmol Soc 2007;105:594–615.

56. Cabrera MT, Freedman SF, Kiely AE, et al. Combining ROPtool measurements of vascular tortuosity and width to quantify plus disease in retinopathy of prematurity. J AAPOS 2011;15(1):40–4.

57. Bullitt E, Gerig G, Pizer SM, et al. Measuring tortuosity of the intracerebral vasculature from MRA images. IEEE Trans Med Imaging 2003;22(9):1163–71.

58. Aylward S, Pizer S, Eberly D, et al. Intensity Ridge and Widths for Tubular Object Segmentation and Description, in MMBIA '96: Proceedings of the 1996 Workshop on Mathematical Methods in Biomedical Image Analysis (MMBIA '96), Washington, DC, USA, 1996. p. 131.

59. Ng J, Clay ST, Barman SA, et al. Maximum likelihood estimation of vessel parameters from scale space analysis. Image Vis Comput 2010;28:55–63.

60. Wilson CM, Cocker KD, Moseley M, et al. Computerized analysis of retinal blood vessel width and tortuosity in eyes at risk for retinopathy of prematurity. Invest Ophthalmol Vis Sci 2008;49:3577–85.

61. Shah DN, Wilson CM, Ying GS, et al. Semiautomated digital image analysis of posterior pole vessels in retinopathy of prematurity. J AAPOS 2009;5:504–6.

62. Ghodasra DH, Karp KA, Ying GS, et al. Risk stratification of preplus retinopathy of prematurity by semi-automated analysis of digital images. Arch Ophthalmol 2010;128(6):719–23.

63. Wilson CM. Classification and automated detection of the retinal vessels of premature infants with and without retinopathy of prematurity [PhD Thesis]. London, UK: City University; 2009.

64. Shah DN, Wilson CM, Ying GS, et al. Comparison of expert graders to computer-assisted image analysis of the retina in retinopathy of prematurity. Br J Ophthalmol 2011;95(10):1442–5.

65. Chiang MF, Gelman R, Martinez-Perez ME, et al. Image analysis for ROP diagnosis. J AAPOS 2009;13:438–45.

66. Wittenberg LA, Jonsson NJ, Chan RV, et al. Computer-based image analysis for plus disease and pre plus disease in ROP. J Pediatr Ophthalmol Strabismus 2012;49:11–9.

67. Wilson C, Theodoru M, Cocker KD, et al. The temporal retinal vessel angle and infants born preterm. Br J Ophthalmol 2006;90(6):702–4.

68. Wong K, Ng J, Ells A, et al. The temporal and nasal retinal and arteriolar and venular angles in infants born preterm. Br J Ophthalmol 2011;95(12):1723–7.

69. Wilson CM, Wong K, Ng J, et al. Digital image analysis in ROP: a comparison of vessel selection methods. J AAPOS 2012;16(3):223–9.

70. Lofqvist C, Hansen-Pupp I, Anderson E, et al. Validation of a new ROP screening method monitoring longitudinal postnatal weight and insulin-like growth factor 1. Arch Ophthalmol 2009;127(5):622–7.

71. Hellstrom A, Hard AL, Engstrom E, et al. Early weight gain predicts retinopathy in preterm infants: new simple, efficient approach to screening. Pediatrics 2009; 123(4):e638–45.

72. Wu C Vanderveen DK, Hellstrmo A, Lofquist C, et al. Longitudinal postnatal weight measurements for the prediction of retinopathy of prematurity. Arch Ophthalmol 2010;128(4):443–7.

73. Binenbaum G, Ying GS, Quinn G, et al. A clinical prediction model to stratify retinopathy of prematurity risk using postnatal weight gain. Pediatrics 2011;127(3): 607–14.
74. Ells A, Guernsey DL, Wallace K, et al. Severe retinopathy of prematurity associated with FZD4 mutations. Ophthalmic Genet 2010;31(1):37–43.
75. Hiraoka M, Bernstein DM, Trese MT, et al. Insertion and deletion mutations in the dinucleotide repeat region of the Norrie disease gene in patients with advanced retinopathy of prematurity. J Hum Genet 2001;46:178–81.
76. Committee for the Classification of Retinopathy of Prematurity. An international classification of retinopathy of prematurity. Br J Ophthalmol 1984;68:690–7.
77. A Second International Committee for the Classification of Retinopathy of Prematurity. The International Classification of Retinopathy of Prematurity - Revisited. Arch Ophthalmol 2005;123:991–9.
78. Early Treatment for Retinopathy of Prematurity Cooperative Group. Revised indications for the treatment of retinopathy of prematurity: results of the Early Treatment for Retinopathy of Prematurity randomized trial. Arch Ophthalmol 2003; 121(12):1684–94.
79. Sociedad Argentina de Pediatria. Recommendations for retinopathy screening in at-risk populations. Arch Argent Pediatr 2008;106:71–6 [in Spanish].
80. Gobierno de Chile. Guia clinica: retinopatia del prematurio. 2005. Available at: http://www.redsalud.gov.ck/archiveos/guiasges/RetinopatiaPrematuorRMayo10.pdf. Accessed January 1, 2013.

Algorithms for the Prediction of Retinopathy of Prematurity Based on Postnatal Weight Gain

Gil Binenbaum, MD, MSCE

KEYWORDS

• Infant • Nomogram • Prediction model • Retinopathy of prematurity • Risk model

KEY POINTS

• Slow postnatal growth is a surrogate measure for low serum insulin-like growth factor 1, which is an important risk factor for severe retinopathy of prematurity (ROP).
• Risk models that consider postnatal weight gain, along with birth weight and gestational age, include WINROP, ROPScore, and CHOP ROP.
• These models predict severe ROP with much greater specificity than current ROP screening guidelines.
• Two important limitations are study sample size and poor generalizability in countries with developing neonatal care systems.
• Postnatal growth-based models have great potential to reduce the number of diagnostic ROP examinations being performed.

INTRODUCTION

Prognostic statistical models allow clinicians to predict a patient's risk of developing a specific medical outcome.[1] Although not typically described in such terms, current retinopathy of prematurity (ROP) screening criteria are a simple prediction model with 2 dichotomized (yes or no) predictors, birth weight (BW) and gestational age at birth (GA). A need for examinations is determined by the degree of prematurity at birth by using 2 cutoff levels, and other risk factors are not considered in a systematic fashion. For example, in the United States, babies with either BW <1501 g or GA ≤30 weeks receive examinations.[2] A priority is placed on avoiding blindness in even a single child, and this screening model has high sensitivity (it catches almost all cases of severe ROP), but it is not specific (most examined infants do not develop severe ROP). In fact, less than 5% of infants examined require laser surgery, based on multiple large US,[3–6] Canadian,[7] and UK[8,9] studies.

Division of Ophthalmology, The Children's Hospital of Philadelphia, 34th Street and Civic Center Boulevard, Philadelphia, PA 19104, USA
E-mail address: binenbaum@email.chop.edu

Clin Perinatol 40 (2013) 261–270
http://dx.doi.org/10.1016/j.clp.2013.02.004   perinatology.theclinics.com
0095-5108/13/$ – see front matter © 2013 Elsevier Inc. All rights reserved.

GROWTH, INSULIN-LIKE GROWTH FACTOR-1, AND ROP

In an effort to improve this specificity, postnatal growth-based ROP risk models have been developed. The models are based on groundbreaking work by Smith, Hellstrom, Lofqvist, and colleagues, who have provided the current understanding of the pathophysiology underlying ROP.

ROP develops in 2 phases, a hypoxic preclinical phase, during which slow postnatal growth can be used to predict risk, and a subsequent proliferative clinical phase. These phases result from alterations in serum insulin-like growth factor-1 (IGF-1), a somatic growth factor, and retinal vascular endothelial growth factor (VEGF), a hypoxia-induced vasoproliferative factor necessary for normal retinal vascular development.[10] Serum IGF-1 decreases with premature birth from loss of maternal sources and poor endogenous production.[11–14] Importantly, IGF-1 plays a permissive role in VEGF-induced retinal vascular growth.[15,16] Therefore, low serum IGF-1 hinders retinal vessel development, with localized hypoxia and VEGF accumulation, as metabolic demands increase within the developing retina. With increasing age and size, endogenous production of IGF-1 increases, permitting VEGF activity, and proliferative retinopathy develops.

Much laboratory work supports this model.[10,15–21] Clinically, multiple investigators have demonstrated that both prolonged early IGF-1 deficits and slow postnatal weight gain are associated with a higher risk of subsequent severe ROP.[11,22–30] Levels of serum IGF-1 correlate with fetal and postnatal growth, so postnatal growth is a good surrogate measure for serum IGF-1.[12,14,31–33] In addition, weight measurements are simple, quick, cheap, and routinely collected, whereas IGF-1 assays are costly and require blood, a laboratory, and processing time.

POSTNATAL GROWTH ROP MODELS

Specific postnatal growth-based ROP predictive models are discussed later in this article. In evaluating these models, it is most useful to consider their performance with regard to sensitivity for detecting severe ROP and the reduction in children requiring eye examinations that would have resulted from their use, which is a more clinically intuitive measure than specificity. Severe ROP has been variably defined as Early Treatment of ROP Study type 1 ROP, treated ROP, or stage 3 ROP in the studies.

All 3 models use weight gain as a measure of postnatal growth and consider BW and GA in the determination of risk of ROP along with growth. BW and GA are still the most significant risk factors for ROP in countries with highly developed neonatal intensive care unit systems.[3–7,9,34–37] The smaller and younger an infant was at birth, the greater the risk of ROP and severity of ROP. Likely pathophysiologic correlates include the degree of retinal vascular immaturity and low postnatal endogenous production of serum IGF-1. However, this predictive information is lost by using only BW and GA cutoff levels. Treating BW and GA as continuous or ordinal variables addresses this issue, but then another factor, such as slow postnatal growth, must be introduced to identify higher BW and GA infants at risk for severe ROP.

With regard to additional risk factors, current screening guidelines do include an unstable clinical course, as judged by the neonatologist as criteria by which to examine larger infants. However, in practice, postnatal factors are not considered in a systematic fashion, even though multiple other risk factors for ROP have been described, such as excessive supplemental oxygen, necrotizing enterocolitis, intraventricular hemorrhage, anemia, apnea, sepsis, and blood transfusions.[6,35,38–44] Based on the studies mentioned in later discussion, it is hypothesized that most such factors may act via a common pathway, by lowering levels of serum IGF-1, and may be captured in a predictive model simply by considering postnatal weight gain. Supplemental oxygen is an important exception, particularly in countries with developing neonatal care systems, whereby higher BW and GA infants may develop severe ROP via a pathophysiologic mechanism unrelated to low serum IGF-1. The limited potential for weight gain ROP models to be used in such infants is a critical issue discussed later.

WINROP

On the basis of their work on IGF-1 and ROP, Lofqvist and colleagues[22] developed a computer-based ROP risk algorithm named WINROP to detect slowdowns in postnatal weight gain, predict severe ROP, and greatly reduce the number of infants requiring examinations.[45–47] WINROP uses a cumulative-deviations statistical approach in multiple steps: each week the infant's actual weight is compared with an expected growth curve of infants who developed no or mild ROP; the differences or deviations between the expected weight and the actual weight are accumulated from week to week; and when these cumulative deviations surpass a level of threshold alarm, the risk of severe ROP is categorized using levels of dichotomized cutoff for BW, GA, and alarm timing to determine a need for eye examinations.

WINROP demonstrated very high sensitivity for detecting severe ROP in retrospective studies: 100% in a Swedish cohort of 353 infants, reducing infants who would have received examinations by 76%[25]; 100% in a Boston cohort of 318 infants, reducing infants who need examinations by 75%[29]; and most recently decreasing slightly to 98.6% in a larger, multicenter US and Canadian cohort of 1706 infants.[48] When WINROP was studied in countries with developing neonatal intensive care unit systems, however, the sensitivity decreased further: 91% in a Brazilian cohort of 366 infants,[49] and 55% (85% if GA <32 weeks, 5% if GA ≥32 weeks) in a Mexican cohort of 352 infants.[50]

The WINROP algorithm involves complex calculations, which have limited transparency for the user. However, the developers have created a Web-based application (www.winrop.com) that permits the user to enter BW, GA, and weight measurements, allows tracking of multiple infants, and provides a simple indication of low-risk or high-risk status for developing site-threatening ROP. The authors suggest that WINROP be used as "an adjunct to and not a replacement for standard ophthalmological screening."[48] They describe abbreviated examination schedules for low-risk infants, as opposed to no examinations at all.[48]

ROPSCORE

Eckert and colleagues[51] recently developed a less complex model named ROPScore. The model consists of a logistic regression equation, which is used to calculate risk only once per child, using an Excel spreadsheet. The model includes continuous rather than dichotomized terms for BW and GA, weight gain at a single time point (6 weeks postnatal age) as a proportion of BW, and dichotomous terms for blood transfusion and use of oxygen in mechanical ventilation during the first 6 weeks of life. Assuming a specific level of cut off for low or high risk, ROPScore had a sensitivity of 98% and specificity of 56% for treatment-requiring ROP in a development cohort of 474 Brazilian infants.[51] Additional studies are underway. As with WINROP, the authors suggest that ROPScore not be used to determine overall screening criteria but rather to reduce the frequency of examinations in low-risk infants.[51]

PINT ROP AND CHOP ROP

Binenbaum and colleagues[30] developed a simpler logistic regression-based model named PINT ROP. Prospectively collected data from 367 infants with BW <1000 g in the Premature Infants in Need of Transfusion (PINT) randomized controlled trial were used to develop a model containing terms only for BW, GA, and daily rate of weight gain, which was calculated from the current and prior week's weight measurements. The equation is calculated on a weekly basis, and if the predicted risk of ROP is greater than a level of cut point, examinations are indicated and the equation does not need to be recalculated. In this manner, PINT ROP had 100% sensitivity for treated ROP, while reducing the number of infants requiring examinations by 30% in the high-risk cohort.[30]

Of note, numerous additional candidate predictors were evaluated, including ethnicity, perinatal and postnatal comorbidities, and medical and surgical interventions. All these factors dropped out in multivariate analyses,[30] supporting the hypothesis that many previously described risk factors for ROP act through a common pathway, by affecting levels of IGF-1, and are therefore captured through weight measurements.

The PINT ROP cohort was at high risk for ROP. Therefore, the investigators applied the same modeling approach to a low-risk cohort more representative of current US ROP screening criteria (BW <1501 g) to develop an updated model called CHOP ROP.[52] Among 524 infants, the model had 100% sensitivity for type 1 ROP, while reducing the number of infants requiring examinations by 49%. If the risk cutoff was raised to miss 1 infant requiring laser, the reduction in examinations was 79%, suggesting a tradeoff that might be explored further. There was a small (3%) advantage to using daily versus weekly weight measurements. Paper nomograms to simplify use of the models were created based on the PINT ROP model and updated with the CHOP ROP model (**Fig. 1**), but the authors stressed that further studies are needed before clinical use.[30,52]

MODEL DEVELOPMENT AND COMPLEXITY

The creation of a usable clinical prediction model is a stepwise process.[1] First, a development study is undertaken, containing as large a sample size as possible to avoid overfitting of the model.[1,53] Overfitting may occur when the complexity of the model is high relative to the number of outcome events (cases of severe ROP) in the cohort, and the model effectively describes random error rather than a true association. Such a model will not perform well in a new group of patients. Second, the model must be validated in new patients and, if necessary, updated, preferably using both the original and new datasets.[1,54,55] Model updating may involve adjusting the model coefficients or even adding new variables if necessary.[55] In the case of the CHOP ROP model, the study cohort had a significantly different risk profile than the PINT ROP cohort, so the model coefficients and alarm cut point needed to be adjusted.

The final step is to evaluate the impact of the model in clinical use.[1,56] Successful implementation of a clinical predictive model requires physician acceptance, which depends on transparency, ease of use, and in this case confidence that no cases of severe ROP will be missed.[56] Transparency and ease of use relate to model complexity, whereas confidence relates most directly to the precision of the point estimate of sensitivity of the model for predicting severe ROP. A cumulative-deviations model is relatively more complex and to some degree lacks transparency with regard to the calculations being performed to determine risk. The process becomes more

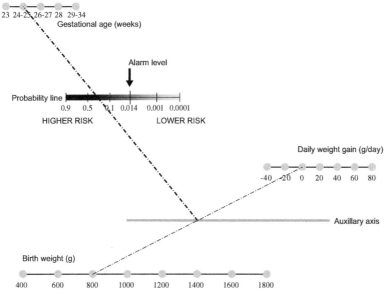

Fig. 1. Sample nomogram to predict the risk of severe ROP based on the CHOP ROP model. A straight line is drawn between the values for birth weight and daily rate of weight gain. The intersection of this line with the gray auxiliary axis is then connected to the value for GA. The intersection of this second line with the probability line provides the predicted probability of severe ROP. If the risk is greater than 0.014, eye examinations are indicated. NOTE: This nomogram requires further validation and is not intended for clinical use at this time. (*From* Binenbaum G, Ying GS, Quinn GE, et al. The CHOP postnatal weight gain, birth weight, and gestaional age retinopathy of prematurity risk model. Arch Ophthalmol 2012;130(12):1560–5; with permission.)

user-friendly with the use of a Web-based application.[22,23,25] A logistic regression equation-based model provides a simpler calculation of risk, and it can be represented as a paper nomogram, which does not require any calculation to be performed (see **Fig. 1**).

SAMPLE SIZE: AN IMPORTANT LIMITATION

Despite studies in cohorts ranging from 300 to 1700 infants, sample size remains a limiting factor. Although a point estimate of sensitivity of 100% has been reported, the confidence interval (CI) around that point estimate is likely too wide for clinicians to have confidence that infants with severe ROP would not be missed. The reason is that the width of the CI is driven by the number of cases of severe ROP, not the overall number of infants. For example, the CHOP ROP study involved 524 infants, but only 20 infants had severe ROP, so whereas the sensitivity was 100%, the 95% CI was 84% to 100%. Even in the most recent, multicenter WINROP study, which involved 1706 infants and reported a sensitivity of 98.6%, the CI was only 96.7% to 100%.

To have sufficient confidence in a model to justify its use for primary all-or-none screening decisions, the lower boundary of the CI arguably should be much higher, perhaps greater than 99%, which would require a dataset with hundreds of cases of ROP. Therefore, it may be best to conservatively consider these studies as still in the developmental stage, and only once that high degree of precision of sensitivity (very narrow CI) is obtained would subsequent validation and updating studies be undertaken. Larger studies might also identify confounding medical factors, the presence of which would default an infant to receive eye examinations. However, alternative perspectives and approaches may be considered. Rather than replacing current screening guidelines, a model may be used alongside current guidelines, changing examination frequency or timing based on predicted risk. WINROP has been used in Sweden in this fashion, based on repeatedly high sensitivity demonstrated across multiple WINROP studies.[48] Alternatively, a sensitivity of less than 100% might be acceptable under some circumstances, such as when ophthalmologic resources are limited and must be rationed. Finally, a model's alarm level could be lowered to more confidently ensure 100% sensitivity, while accepting a decrease in specificity. This approach could work well in a multitiered screening approach together with telemedicine, once both modalities have been sufficiently validated: the risk model determines which infants require fundus photographs, and photographic grading determines which infants require eye examination by an ophthalmologist.

GENERALIZABILITY: A SECOND IMPORTANT LIMITATION

There are several reasons a predictive model may behave poorly in new patients, including the methods used to design the model and differences in health care systems and patient characteristics.[54] There is good evidence that the generalizability of models such as WINROP and CHOP ROP to countries where higher BW and GA infants develop severe ROP will be limited, and that separate model development studies need to be performed in such populations. When WINROP was applied to a Brazilian cohort, it demonstrated less than 90% sensitivity,[49] and when it was applied to a Mexican cohort, sensitivity was only 55%.[50] ROPScore was developed in Brazil, and model performance was higher.[51] However, additional terms for blood transfusion and oxygen supplementation are included in the model,[51] and performance across multiple settings still must be assessed, as there is high variability in ROP risk profile across neonatal centers in the country, even within the same city.[57]

The poor performance of postnatal weight gain ROP models in countries with developing neonatal care systems may be related to differences in ROP pathophysiology, particularly in older GA infants. At older postmenstrual ages, endogenous production of IGF-1 has already increased, so that low IGF-1 may play less of a role in the pathogenesis of severe ROP. Rather, ROP in such infants might be driven primarily by high oxygen exposure, which causes inhibition of VEGF and retinal blood vessel destruction, as it does in oxygen-induced animal models of ROP. This hypothesis is supported by the dramatic difference in the performance of WINROP among Mexican infants with GA <32 weeks (85% sensitivity) and GA $\geq$32 weeks (5% sensitivity).

BENEFITS AND FUTURE STUDIES

Improved ROP risk assessment could have broad-reaching benefits in neonatology, ophthalmology, and public health. Revised ROP screening guidelines might reduce both the number of children requiring stressful diagnostic eye examinations and the frequency of examinations for lower risk infants. Professional and infrastructure resources may be better allocated to high-risk infants, particularly in areas and countries with limited resources, where better targeted resources could lower the burden of blindness caused by ROP. Tiered approaches, combining a growth-based risk model with telemedicine assessments, might further improve the efficiency of screening. In general, the cost effectiveness of ROP diagnostic examinations would be increased.

Postnatal weight-gain–based ROP prediction models have great potential to influence the clinical management of ROP. Further development, validation, and clinical impact studies across multiple international settings can and should be pursued, but there are no set epidemiologic rules by which to determine when sufficient validation has been achieved to safely use a clinical prediction model; criteria depend on the clinical context.[55] ROP screening involves high-stakes decisions, and perhaps model validation and updating will best be viewed as an ongoing process. The studies discussed have established proof of concept. If even larger development and validation studies continue to demonstrate very high sensitivity for predicting severe ROP, then the research objective will shift toward simply maximizing the predictive value of the data on which ROP screening guidelines are based. Retrospective pooling of datasets by investigators and an ongoing prospective data registry would permit a model to be updated in an ongoing fashion and maximize the use of available data. This type of collaborative approach would best ensure that all infants at risk for site-threatening ROP undergo diagnostic eye examinations, while the potential benefits of postnatal growth based ROP models are realized.

REFERENCES

1. Moons KG, Royston P, Vergouwe Y, et al. Prognosis and prognostic research: what, why, and how? BMJ 2009;338:1317–20.
2. Fierson WM, American Academy of Pediatrics Section on Ophthalmology, American Academy of Ophthalmology, et al. Screening examination of premature infants for retinopathy of prematurity. Pediatrics 2013;131(1):189–95.
3. The natural ocular outcome of premature birth and retinopathy. Status at 1 year. Cryotherapy for Retinopathy of Prematurity Cooperative Group. Arch Ophthalmol 1994;112(7):903–12.
4. Palmer EA, Flynn JT, Hardy RJ, et al. Incidence and early course of retinopathy of prematurity. The Cryotherapy for Retinopathy of Prematurity Cooperative Group. Ophthalmology 1991;98(11):1628–40.
5. Early Treatment For Retinopathy Of Prematurity Cooperative Group. Revised indications for the treatment of retinopathy of prematurity: results of the early treatment for retinopathy of prematurity randomized trial. Arch Ophthalmol 2003; 121(12):1684–94.
6. Chiang MF, Arons RR, Flynn JT, et al. Incidence of retinopathy of prematurity from 1996 to 2000: analysis of a comprehensive New York state patient database. Ophthalmology 2004;111(7):1317–25.
7. Lee SK, Normand C, McMillan D, et al. Evidence for changing guidelines for routine screening for retinopathy of prematurity. Arch Pediatr Adolesc Med 2001;155(3):387–95.
8. Haines L, Fielder AR, Scrivener R, et al. Retinopathy of prematurity in the UK I: the organisation of services for screening and treatment. Eye (Lond) 2002;16(1): 33–8.
9. Royal College of Paediatrics and Child Health RCoO, British Association of Perinatal Medicine. UK Retinopathy of Prematurity Guideline May 2008. [PDF]. UK Retinopathy of Prematurity Guideline. 2008. Available at: http://www.rcophth. ac.uk/core/core_picker/download.asp?id=180&filetitle=UK+Retinopathy+of+ Prematurity+Guideline+May+2008. Accessed September 17, 2012.
10. Pierce EA, Foley ED, Smith LE. Regulation of vascular endothelial growth factor by oxygen in a model of retinopathy of prematurity. Arch Ophthalmol 1996;114(10): 1219–28.

11. Hellstrom A, Engstrom E, Hard AL, et al. Postnatal serum insulin-like growth factor I deficiency is associated with retinopathy of prematurity and other complications of premature birth. Pediatrics 2003;112(5):1016–20.
12. Langford K, Nicolaides K, Miell JP. Maternal and fetal insulin-like growth factors and their binding proteins in the second and third trimesters of human pregnancy. Hum Reprod 1998;13(5):1389–93.
13. Lassarre C, Hardouin S, Daffos F, et al. Serum insulin-like growth factors and insulin-like growth factor binding proteins in the human fetus. Relationships with growth in normal subjects and in subjects with intrauterine growth retardation. Pediatr Res 1991;29(3):219–25.
14. Lineham JD, Smith RM, Dahlenburg GW, et al. Circulating insulin-like growth factor I levels in newborn premature and full-term infants followed longitudinally. Early Hum Dev 1986;13(1):37–46.
15. Smith LE, Shen W, Perruzzi C, et al. Regulation of vascular endothelial growth factor-dependent retinal neovascularization by insulin-like growth factor-1 receptor. Nat Med 1999;5(12):1390–5.
16. Hellstrom A, Perruzzi C, Ju M, et al. Low IGF-I suppresses VEGF-survival signaling in retinal endothelial cells: direct correlation with clinical retinopathy of prematurity. Proc Natl Acad Sci U S A 2001;98(10):5804–8.
17. Aiello LP, Pierce EA, Foley ED, et al. Suppression of retinal neovascularization in vivo by inhibition of vascular endothelial growth factor (VEGF) using soluble VEGF-receptor chimeric proteins. Proc Natl Acad Sci U S A 1995;92(23):10457–61.
18. Alon T, Hemo I, Itin A, et al. Vascular endothelial growth factor acts as a survival factor for newly formed retinal vessels and has implications for retinopathy of prematurity. Nat Med 1995;1(10):1024–8.
19. Pierce EA, Avery RL, Foley ED, et al. Vascular endothelial growth factor/vascular permeability factor expression in a mouse model of retinal neovascularization. Proc Natl Acad Sci U S A 1995;92(3):905–9.
20. Robinson GS, Pierce EA, Rook SL, et al. Oligodeoxynucleotides inhibit retinal neovascularization in a murine model of proliferative retinopathy. Proc Natl Acad Sci U S A 1996;93(10):4851–6.
21. Shih SC, Ju M, Liu N, et al. Selective stimulation of VEGFR-1 prevents oxygen-induced retinal vascular degeneration in retinopathy of prematurity. J Clin Invest 2003;112(1):50–7.
22. Lofqvist C, Andersson E, Sigurdsson J, et al. Longitudinal postnatal weight and insulin-like growth factor I measurements in the prediction of retinopathy of prematurity. Arch Ophthalmol 2006;124(12):1711–8.
23. Lofqvist C, Hansen-Pupp I, Andersson E, et al. Validation of a new retinopathy of prematurity screening method monitoring longitudinal postnatal weight and insulinlike growth factor I. Arch Ophthalmol 2009;127(5):622–7.
24. Perez-Munuzuri A, Fernandez-Lorenzo J, Couce-Pico M, et al. Serum levels of IGF1 are a useful predictor of retinopathy of prematurity. Acta Paediatr 2010;99(4):519–25.
25. Hellstrom A, Hard AL, Engstrom E, et al. Early weight gain predicts retinopathy in preterm infants: new, simple, efficient approach to screening. Pediatrics 2009;123(4):e638–45.
26. Wallace DK, Kylstra JA, Phillips SJ, et al. Poor postnatal weight gain: a risk factor for severe retinopathy of prematurity. J AAPOS 2000;4(6):343–7.
27. Fortes Filho JB, Bonomo PP, Maia M, et al. Weight gain measured at 6 weeks after birth as a predictor for severe retinopathy of prematurity: study with 317 very low

birth weight preterm babies. Graefes Arch Clin Exp Ophthalmol 2009;247(6): 831–6.

28. Villegas-Becerril E, González-Fernández R, Perula-Torres L, et al. IGF-1, VEGF, and bFGF as predictive factors for the onset of Retinopathy of Prematurity (ROP). Arch Soc Esp Oftalmol 2006;81:641–6 [in Spanish].

29. Wu C, Vanderveen DK, Hellstrom A, et al. Longitudinal postnatal weight measurements for the prediction of retinopathy of prematurity. Arch Ophthalmol 2010; 128(4):443–7.

30. Binenbaum G, Ying GS, Quinn GE, et al. A clinical prediction model to stratify retinopathy of prematurity risk using postnatal weight gain. Pediatrics 2011;127(3): e607–14.

31. Ahmad I, Zaldivar F, Iwanaga K, et al. Inflammatory and growth mediators in growing preterm infants. J Pediatr Endocrinol Metab 2007;20(3):387–96.

32. Grimberg A, Cohen P. Role of insulin-like growth factors and their binding proteins in growth control and carcinogenesis. J Cell Physiol 2000;183(1):1–9.

33. Hikino S, Ihara K, Yamamoto J, et al. Physical growth and retinopathy in preterm infants: involvement of IGF-I and GH. Pediatr Res 2001;50(6):732–6.

34. Duhaime AC, Alario AJ, Lewander WJ, et al. Head injury in very young children: mechanisms, injury types, and ophthalmologic findings in 100 hospitalized patients younger than 2 years of age. Pediatrics 1992;90(2 Pt 1):179–85.

35. Lucey JF, Dangman B. A reexamination of the role of oxygen in retrolental fibroplasia. Pediatrics 1984;73(1):82–96.

36. Ng YK, Fielder AR, Shaw DE, et al. Epidemiology of retinopathy of prematurity. Lancet 1988;2(8622):1235–8.

37. Schaffer DB, Palmer EA, Plotsky DF, et al. Prognostic factors in the natural course of retinopathy of prematurity. The Cryotherapy for Retinopathy of Prematurity Cooperative Group. Ophthalmology 1993;100(2):230–7.

38. Hutchinson AK, O'Neil JW, Morgan EN, et al. Retinopathy of prematurity in infants with birth weights greater than 1250 grams. J AAPOS 2003;7(3):190–4.

39. Yanovitch TL, Siatkowski RM, McCaffree M, et al. Retinopathy of prematurity in infants with birth weight>or=1250 grams-incidence, severity, and screening guideline cost-analysis. J AAPOS 2006;10(2):128–34.

40. Gilbert C. Retinopathy of prematurity: a global perspective of the epidemics, population of babies at risk and implications for control. Early Hum Dev 2008; 84(2):77–82.

41. Mohamed S, Schaa K, Cooper ME, et al. Genetic contributions to the development of retinopathy of prematurity. Pediatr Res 2009;65(2):193–7.

42. Ben Sira I, Nissenkorn I, Kremer I. Retinopathy of prematurity. Surv Ophthalmol 1988;33(1):1–16.

43. Fielder AR, Shaw DE, Robinson J, et al. Natural history of retinopathy of prematurity: a prospective study. Eye (Lond) 1992;6(Pt 3):233–42.

44. Shohat M, Reisner SH, Krikler R, et al. Retinopathy of prematurity: incidence and risk factors. Pediatrics 1983;72(2):159–63.

45. Frisen M. Statistical surveillance: optimality and methods. Int Stat Rev 2003;71(2): 403–34.

46. Roberts SW. A comparison of some control chart procedures. Technometrics 1966;8(3):411–30, 435.

47. Shiryaev A. On optimum methods in quickest detection problems. Theor Probab Appl 1963;8(1):22–46.

48. Wu C, Lofqvist C, Smith LE, et al. Importance of early postnatal weight gain for normal retinal angiogenesis in very preterm infants: a multicenter study analyzing

weight velocity deviations for the prediction of retinopathy of prematurity. Arch Ophthalmol 2012;130(8):992–9.

49. Hard AL, Lofqvist C, Fortes Filho JB, et al. Predicting proliferative retinopathy in a Brazilian population of preterm infants with the screening algorithm WINROP. Arch Ophthalmol 2010;128(11):1432–6.

50. Zepeda-Romero LC, Hard AL, Gomez-Ruiz LM, et al. Prediction of retinopathy of prematurity using the screening algorithm WINROP in a Mexican population of preterm infants. Arch Ophthalmol 2012;130(6):720–3.

51. Eckert GU, Fortes Filho JB, Maia M, et al. A predictive score for retinopathy of prematurity in very low birth weight preterm infants. Eye (Lond) 2012;26(3):400–6.

52. Binenbaum G, Ying GS, Quinn GE, et al. The CHOP postnatal weight gain, birth weight, and gestational age retinopathy of prematurity risk model. Arch Ophthalmol 2012;130(12):1560–5.

53. Royston P, Moons KG, Altman DG, et al. Prognosis and prognostic research: developing a prognostic model. BMJ 2009;338:b604.

54. Altman DG, Vergouwe Y, Royston P, et al. Prognosis and prognostic research: validating a prognostic model. BMJ 2009;338:b605.

55. Moons KG, Altman DG, Vergouwe Y, et al. Prognosis and prognostic research: application and impact of prognostic models in clinical practice. BMJ 2009; 338:b606.

56. Wyatt JC, Altman DG. Commentary: prognostic models: clinically useful or quickly forgotten. Br Med J 1995;311:1539–41.

57. Zin AA, Moreira ME, Bunce C, et al. Retinopathy of prematurity in 7 neonatal units in Rio de Janeiro: screening criteria and workload implications. Pediatrics 2010; 126(2):e410–7.

Optical Coherence Tomography in Retinopathy of Prematurity

Looking Beyond the Vessels

Ramiro S. Maldonado, MD[a], Cynthia A. Toth, MD[a,b],*

KEYWORDS

- Optical coherence tomography • Age-customized OCT imaging approach
- Retinopathy of prematurity • Macular edema of prematurity • Plus disease

KEY POINTS

- Optical Coherence Tomography (OCT) is a relatively new imaging technology capable of imaging ocular structures in cross section at high resolution. Utilizing this imaging modality one can visualize the retina, choroid and optic nerve at microscopic level.
- An age-customized approach to perform OCT in neonates, infants and children is necessary to improve image quality and efficacy. Time per imaging session is also reduced.
- OCT can provide sub-clinical information.
- OCT can show the in-vivo maturation of the human fovea at the cellular and sub-cellular level.
- Spectral Domain OCT is a faster OCT modality that allows acquisition of retinal volumetric scans. Other new SDOCT modalities such as enhanced depth imaging (EDI) and color doppler are discussed.

OPTICAL COHERENCE TOMOGRAPHY

Background

Optical coherence tomography (OCT) is a diagnostic imaging tool that provides cross-sectional images of the retina. It was first described in 1991 by Huang and colleagues[1] and became commercially available in 1996. Since then, it has improved diagnosis

Funding for this research was provided by The Hartwell Foundation; Research to Prevent Blindness and Grant 1UL1 RR024128-01 from the National Center for Research Resources (NCRR), a component of the National Institutes of Health (NIH); and NIH Roadmap for Medical Research. Dr. Toth receives other research support from Bioptigen.

[a] Department of Ophthalmology, Duke University Medical Center, 2351 Erwin Road, Durham, NC, USA; [b] Department of Biomedical Engineering, Pratt School of Engineering, Duke University, Room 136 Hudson Hall, Box 90281, Durham, NC 27708, USA
* Corresponding author. Duke University Eye Center, 2351 Erwin Road, Suite 103, DARSI Laboratory, Durham, NC 27710.
E-mail address: cynthia.toth@duke.edu

Clin Perinatol 40 (2013) 271–296
http://dx.doi.org/10.1016/j.clp.2013.02.007
0095-5108/13/$ – see front matter © 2013 Elsevier Inc. All rights reserved.

and management of retinal diseases and is considered standard of care in age-related macular degeneration and diabetic retinopathy among other adult retinal diseases.

OCT works by projecting a broadband light into the eye, with the most common commercial systems centered around ~840 nm wavelength. The backscattered light is then combined for comparison with light reflected from a reference arm. The combination of both lights generates an interference signal. As the beam of light sweeps across the retina, these interference patterns are processed to form the cross-sectional images of the living tissue.

The early ophthalmic OCT design was named time domain OCT (TDOCT) because the reference arm moving mirror is translated in time to scan the depth of the retina. Because of this feature, early versions of ophthalmic OCT had limited speed of scan acquisition and limited resolution. TDOCT evolved to what is now known as spectral-domain OCT (SDOCT), an OCT imaging modality that uses a fixed mirror reference arm and analyzes the interference signal based on the wavelength of light. SDOCT became available in 2002, providing better axial image resolution and faster scan acquisition. The use of improved broader bandwidth light sources also improved the lateral resolution (**Table 1**).[2,3] A new OCT modality with even higher speed, swept-source OCT, is currently available in research systems, with promising capabilities of imaging the retina and choroid.[4,5]

OCT Clinical Applications

There are many applications for OCT within the body (eg, skin, major vessels, heart)[6]; however, the first and most extensive use still remains within the eye, for cornea, lens, iridocorneal angle, retina, choroid, and optic nerve. In the retina, OCT has been used most extensively in the diagnosis and management of glaucoma and vitreoretinal diseases (**Table 2**) in older children and adults. In these populations, OCT also plays a major role in providing measurable end points for clinical trials in diseases such as macular degeneration or vitreous traction.[7,8]

Normal Adult Versus Infant Macular SDOCT

SDOCT cross-sectional images of the retina (B-scans) show retinal architecture by providing information on vitreous, retinal, and foveal shape, differentiation of all retinal layers, choroid, and choroid-scleral junction. The particular spatial arrangement of cells and subcellular elements in the retina provides different reflectivity profiles, which often contrast with adjacent layers. In general, nuclear layers appear hyporeflective and axonal and dendrite layers appear hyperreflective, as seen in **Fig. 1**.

Table 1
OCT modalities: technical characteristics

	TDOCT	SDOCT	Swept Source
Signal-to-noise ratio	Low	High	High
Speed	1×	50× to 250×	250× to 1000×
A-scans/s	400	20,000–100,000	100,000–400,000
Motion artifacts	Frequent	Reduced	Reduced
Volumetric scans	No	Yes	Yes
Axial resolution (μm)	>10	<5	5–6
Lateral resolution (μm)	20–30	<10	10–20

Table 2
Vitreoretinal structures and diseases evaluated by OCT

Structure	Disease
Vitreous	Vitreomacular attachment and traction
Preretinal	Epiretinal membranes Neovascularization Fibrovascular tissue
Retina	Macular holes Cystoid macular edema Schisis Swelling/thickening Deformation/folding Atrophy/degeneration Drug toxicity Subretinal fluid Retinal detachments Pigment epithelium detachment Choroidal neovascularization
Optic nerve	Glaucoma Optic nerve malformations Swelling Atrophy

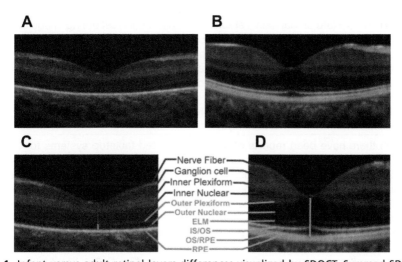

Fig. 1. Infant versus adult retinal layers differences visualized by SDOCT. Summed SDOCT B-scans at the fovea. (*A*) From a 31-week-old PMA premature infant (born at 27 weeks PMA, birth weight 1205 g, ROP zone II, stage 2) and (*B*) from a 23-year-old adult born at term. (*C, D*) are magnified images of (*A, B*), respectively, to show retinal layers in better detail. From inner (*top*) to outer (*bottom*), the layers are nerve fiber layer, ganglion cell layer (GCL), inner plexiform layer (IPL), inner nuclear layer (INL), outer plexiform layer (OPL), outer nuclear layer, external limiting membrane, inner segment (IS) to outer segment (OS), photoreceptor OS, and retinal pigment epithelium (RPE) microvilli, and RPE. Note that the thick IRLs of the neonate (*blue upper vertical line, layers listed in blue*) correspond to thin condensed corresponding layers in the adult and that the thin outer retinal layers of the neonate (*orange lower vertical line*) became thicker layers in the adult eye (*listed in orange; external limiting membrane [ELM], IS/OS, and OS/RPE were not present in the premature fovea*). (*From* Maldonado RS, O'Connell RV, Sarin N, et al. Dynamics of human foveal development after premature birth. Ophthalmology 2011;118(12):2316; with permission.)

As noted on **Fig. 1**, the infant fovea has several differences compared with the adult fovea. This observation led to the first in vivo study of human foveal development using SDOCT,[9] in which SDOCT scans of the fovea were obtained and analyzed from 31 weeks postmenstrual age (PMA) until adulthood, with observations of centrifugal inner retinal layer migration and centripetal outer retinal layer growth in the first months of life in prematurely born infants. Furthermore, with segmentation techniques, the thickness of individual retinal layers has been studied in the prenatal period, showing progressive thinning at the foveal center and thickening on the parafoveal region with increasing age, whereas the inner segment and outer segment thicknesses appear and then increase at the foveal center as the infant grows (**Fig. 2**).[9,10]

An important feature of SDOCT is the capability of producing two-dimensional maps and three-dimensional volumes from the numerous captured B-scans (**Fig. 3**). This feature aids in localization of structures or pathologic processes within the retina[11] and is particularly useful for finding the fovea when the patient does not fixate.

Need for SDOCT in the Pediatric Population

More than 1.4 million children are blind, and millions visually impaired worldwide.[12] Ninety percent of blind children receive no schooling, representing one-third of the economic cost of blindness. In the United States, it is estimated that more than 50,000 children are legally blind, with retinal diseases being the leading ocular cause after cortical blindness.[13]

Most SDOCT systems were designed as tabletop units for adults and cooperative patients able to fixate or maintain a stable position in a chin rest during image capture. We believe that there is a need not only for SDOCT systems designed for the pediatric population but also for an imaging methodology designed for the small pediatric eye. Along with new portable devices, an adequate methodology is needed to capture and interpret SDOCT in infants, neonates, and children.

OPTIMIZING OCT FOR INFANTS, ADULTS, AND CHILDREN
Equipment: Handheld and Portable Systems

Although there have been reports of using unmounted tabletop systems for OCT in infants,[14,15] we believe that this is not the ideal methodology, because the delicate neonates and infants may be exposed to unnecessary discomfort and manipulation, in addition to having to be taken out of their cribs for imaging with large systems. It is useful to have OCT systems designed to be as portable as possible to limit the impact on an infant in an intensive care setting.

Two portable SDOCT systems are commercially available in the United States. Bioptigen (Durham, NC) has an SDOCT system mounted into a rolling cart, making it portable to different scenarios within a medical center (**Fig. 4**). The handheld scanner is small, weighs less than 0.9 kg (2 pounds) and fits into the imager's hand (see **Fig. 4**). This system has been cleared by the US Food and Drug Administration for imaging eyes of infants and children. Optovue (Freemont, CA) has an approximately 2.3-kg (5-pound) scanner head used on an armature for imaging patients in the supine position. In addition, this device has a fundus camera to allow imager guidance to the area of interest. Both systems have been used by different groups across several countries.[16–18]

Developing an Age-Customized Protocol

Optic properties of the infant eye

There are several anatomic and optic differences in the premature eye compared with the adult eye. Dramatic ocular growth occurs during the latter months of preterm

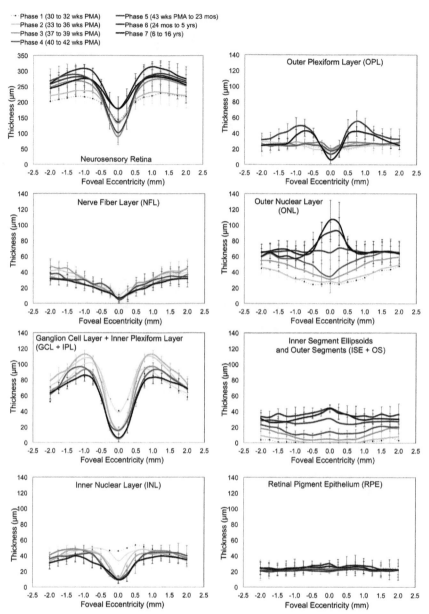

Fig. 2. Retinal layer thickness redistribution during foveal development quantified by SDOCT image segmentation. Mean retinal layer thicknesses are represented from 30 weeks PMA to 16 years. Premature infants are in phases 1 and 2, phases 3 and 4 include term birth, and children are in phases 5 to 7. The youngest age group (phase 1) is represented by a pale dotted line with increasing color intensity up to the oldest (phase 7), a black line. Standard deviations are plotted as error bars. This figure shows a centrifugal redistribution of inner retinal layers (*box plots on the left*) and centripetal growth at the photoreceptor layers (*box plots on the right*). *From* Vajzovic L, Hendrickson AE, O'Connell RV, et al. Maturation of the human fovea: correlation of spectral-domain optical coherence tomography with histology. Am J Ophthalmol 2012;154(5):782; with permission.

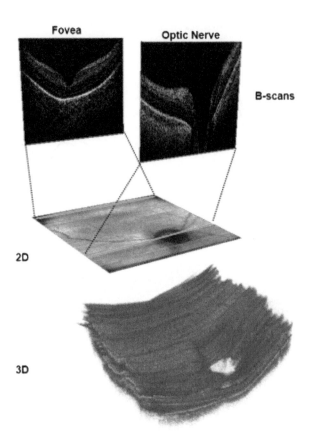

Fig. 3. Two-dimensional (2D) and three-dimensional (3D) images obtained from volumetric SDOCT scans from a 31-week-old PMA infant. Volumetric 6 × 6 mm SDOCT scan from a 31-week-old PMA infant. Sixty B-scans were acquired in less than 4 seconds, with minimal motion detected during acquisition. The foveal and optic nerve B-scans are shown in the top of the figure. By collapsing axially all the pixels from each B-scan, a 2 fundus image (*middle*) comparable with a fundus photo can be obtained. Using volume rendering software, a 3D reconstruction was achieved (*bottom*), showing the optic nerve cup and the retinal surface contour.

development. Investigations with ocular echography have estimated the ocular axial length of the premature infant as 15 mm at 31 weeks PMA and reported the fastest growth to take place from 32 to 52 weeks PMA[19]; during the neonatal period (31–52 weeks PMA), the axial length increases 0.16 mm per week and then slows down to 1 mm per year during the first 2 years of life.[20] The cornea is also steeper and astigmatic in premature infants and the spherically equivalent refraction tends to be myopic, progressing toward hyperopia only after 52 weeks PMA.[21,22] Based on measurements provided by Gordon and Donzis and by Cook and colleagues,[23] we calculated a premature schematic eye model that simplifies the optical power of the ocular structures into a single lens calculation, which is useful in optimizing systems to image the retina (**Table 3**).

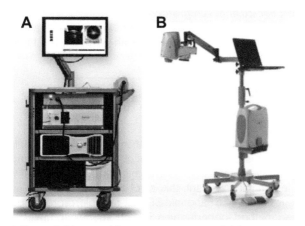

Fig. 4. Commercially available portable SDOCT systems useful for supine imaging. (*A*) Bioptigen Envisu system. 0.9-kg (2-pound) handheld scanner. Speed of 32,000 A-scans per second and 3.3-μm axial resolution for handheld imaging of premature infants to adults. (*B*) Optovue iStand system with a 2.3-kg (5-pound) head scanner supported by an articulating arm, with live en face image for targeting. Speed of 26,000 A-scans per second and a 5-μm axial resolution for supine patient imaging. Product labeling in 2012 for the iVue system with the iStand does not mention pediatric use. (*A: Courtesy of* Bioptigen, Inc., Morrisville, NC; with permission; *B: Courtesy of* Optovue, Inc., Fremont, CA; with permission.)

Table 3
Comparison of schematic eye models for adults, newborns, and premature infants

Schematic Eye Properties	Gullstrand Adult	Benner-Rannets Adult-Modern	Lotmar Newborn[23]	Maldonado et al Premature[24]
Total eye power (D)	58.64	60	84.8	96.54
Eye axial length (mm)	24	24.09	17.49	15.1
Anterior focal length (mm)	−17.055	−16.67	−11.8	−10.35
Posterior focal length (mm)	22.78	22.27	15.74	13.81
Corneal power (D)	43.05	43.08	48.9	55.25
Corneal curvature radius	7.7	7.8	7.26	6.1
Lens power (D)	19.11	20.83	43.4	43.5
Refractive error (D)	1	0	+2.8	−1
Refractive Index				
Air	1	1	1	1
Cornea	1.376	1.377	1.377	1.377
Aqueous	1.336	1336	1.336	1.336
Lens	1.386	1.422	1.43	1.43
Vitreous	1.336	1.336	1.334	1.334

From Maldonado RS, Izatt JA, Sarin N, et al. Optimizing hand-held spectral-domain optical coherence tomography imaging for neonates, infants and children. Invest Ophthalmol Vis Sci 2010;51:2681; with permission.

Justification for an age-customized protocol

If the previously mentioned optic properties are not considered, and SDOCT in neonates or infants is performed as it would be with an adult, the following problems may be encountered (**Fig. 5**A, B):

- Small field of view
- Magnified retinal image
- Image clipping (lateral shadowing by the iris)
- Poor image resolution/clarity

As a consequence, imaging in pediatric patients would remain difficult and inefficient. To correct these issues, imaging protocols need to be customized according to the infant's eye properties based on ocular axial length. Although it would be useful to measure axial length in each infant, this is not often feasible in the nursery. Thus, to address these issues and make handheld SDOCT feasible, reproducible, and efficient, an age-customized method for performing SDOCT image capture in infants has been proposed.[23] This methodology provides adjustments based on the infant's age.

Calculating real scan length on the retina

Smaller eyes produce a magnification effect on the OCT image (see **Fig. 5**A). This situation is primarily a result of the shorter axial length of the eye. A correction is necessary to obtain accurate measurements in the retina. We use the infant versus adult axial length proportion to correct for the lateral magnification: thus, the OCT

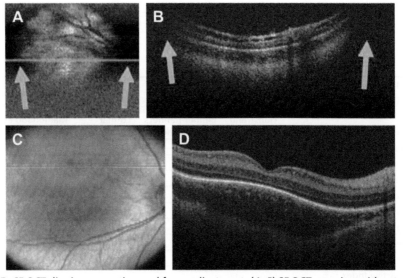

Fig. 5. SDOCT clipping correction and focus adjustment. (*A, B*) SDOCT scanning without age-customized protocol. Severe clipping artifacts (*white arrows*) on the two-dimensional retinal image (*A*) and on the B-scan (*B*) of a 38-week-old PMA infant are noted in addition to poor image quality. (*C, D*) Images were obtained after applying the age-customized protocol. Improved field of view in the retinal image (*C*) and on the B-scan (*D*) with improved image quality. The inner retina in (*B*) shows schisis in an eye with peripheral retinal detachment. The fovea in (*D*) shows persisting inner retinal layers in an older premature infant. (*From* Maldonado RS, Izatt JA, Sarin N, et al. Optimizing hand-held spectral-domain optical coherence tomography imaging for neonates, infants and children. Invest Ophthalmol Vis Sci 2010;51:2682; with permission.)

scan length on the infant retina equals the ratio of infant axial length/adult axial length multiplied by the expected adult OCT lateral scan length.[24] In the example shown in **Fig. 5C** and D, the scan length entered for adult scanning by the OCT system was 11 mm. Because this infant was 38 weeks old PMA (estimated axial length of 16.1 mm), the correct scan length on the infant retina is 7 mm (36% shorter).

Reducing number of A-scans

As explained earlier, the real scan length on the retina of an infant eye is smaller than the scan size set for the adult eye on an OCT system. If the regular presets included with the system software are used, the retina may be exposed to unnecessary light for imaging. Our group proposed adjusting the number of A-scans per B-scan for SDOCT imaging in infant eyes to maintain the same scan density as in adults (**Fig. 6**).

Improving field of view: adjusting the reference arm

The OCT beam has a pivoting point, which should be located at the level of the pupil. In shorter eyes, the pivoting point is displaced anterior to the pupil and thus the peripheral area of the image is clipped as shown in **Fig. 5A** and B. A correction to the reference arm position (index of refraction of the vitreous times the change in axial length of the eye) has been calculated and applied in imaging using the Bioptigen system in premature infants.[24]

The application of this correction provides a wider field of view, as shown in **Fig. 5C** and D.

GENERAL PEDIATRIC SDOCT IMAGING IN THE NEONATAL INTENSIVE CARE UNIT
Step-by-Step Procedure

A step-by-step methodology is proposed, to reduce the time spent imaging, reduce infant discomfort, and produce better imaging results. First, the infant's age in weeks PMA, ocular refraction, and axial length are needed. The axial length and ocular refraction are generally not available but can be estimated based on the infant's age according to biometric studies performed in infant eyes.[20,21] Second, these figures are used to age-adjust the reference arm position, the focus of the lens bore of the system, and

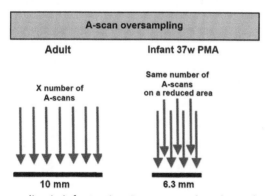

Fig. 6. A-scan oversampling in infant retina. Because scan lengths set for an adult eye project as a shorter scan in the smaller infant eyes, the number of A-scans should be reduced to maintain the same A-scan spacing as in the adult standard eye. Most commercial SDOCT systems come with preset scans for adults, and the same settings should not be applied to infants. An ideal OCT system for infant imaging should provide the imager with the capability of modifying the number of A-scans as desired.

scan parameters such as scan length, number of A-scans, and number of B-scans are entered based on age. Maldonado and colleagues[24] described a step-by-step look-up table convenient for performing all these adjustments.

Once all these steps have been taken, the next step is to position the baby as shown in **Fig. 7** and gently open the eyelids with the tip of the imager's fingers. No lid speculum or anesthetic drops are needed. In some instances, when the baby is restless, the imager can consider using oral sucrose. Although we normally perform SDOCT on the same day of retinopathy of prematurity (ROP) screening when the baby's pupils are dilated, we have performed SDOCT on undilated pupils. In those cases, we found imaging to be more difficult, but we were able to image the fovea and optic nerve with success (**Fig. 8**).

Impact of Applying Age-Customized Settings

In a pilot study applying the previously mentioned methodology in 113 imaging sessions,[24] we reported a decrease in the time per imaging session. An adequate SDOCT image was captured in less than 1 minute in 31% of sessions, 1 to 2 minutes in 26%, and more than 2 minutes in 43%. The average time spent in an imaging session per infant was 11 minutes, including both eyes. An assessment of vital signs during imaging (heart rate, respiratory rate, and oxygen saturation) revealed no change of more than 20% from baseline in 98% of patients. No adverse events were reported by the nurses when we inquired 2 hours after the imaging session occurred.

Limitations and special situations that prevent better imaging results

Overall, this technique seems to be without discomfort for the infant. Most of the time, the infant continues sleeping and seems comfortable. The fact that we do not use a lid speculum or bright illumination such as from a fundus camera or indirect ophthalmoscope seems to help. There are some occasions when the infant seems to be restless or has, for example, a neurologic baseline problem that causes them to be constantly moving, not only their eyes but also their body. Faster low-density scans increase the chance of obtaining useful images of the fovea or optic nerve in the moving infant by reducing the time needed to complete the scans.

With current systems, the maximal area of SDOCT imaging covers typically only zone I (**Fig. 9**). Clipping caused by the pupil also prevents OCT scanning across a

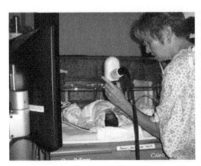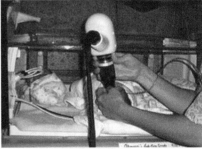

Fig. 7. SDOCT imaging in the neonatal intensive care unit (NICU). Typical SDOCT imaging methodology in the NICU. With the infant lying comfortably in the crib (*left*), the imager gently opens the eyelids with the fingertips and holds the handheld SDOCT scanner over the infant's eyes without touching the infant or the infant's eye (*right*). The weight of the scanner is centered over the imager's hand, and the distal tip of the lens system can be steadied by the fingers holding the eyelids. A second operator operates the software and captures the scans. The scanner and the infant's head could be tilted or moved to acquire the area of interest.

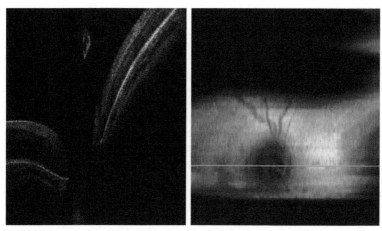

Fig. 8. SDOCT image capturing in an infant with 3 mm pupil dilation. (*Left*) B-scan at the center of the optic nerve without clipping artifacts. (*Right*) Two-dimensional retinal image showing clipping artifacts caused by the pupil and imager/infant motion.

wider field of view, despite the age-customized protocols described earlier. During an imaging session, an experienced imager may be able to obtain more information in the periphery by scanning serially different retinal areas and making a collage of images, which could increase the field of view into zone II. Because of this situation, SDOCT is not typically effective for viewing the vascular-avascular junction.

Another limitation is equipment cost, which may prevent widespread use of this technique at multiple smaller medical centers.

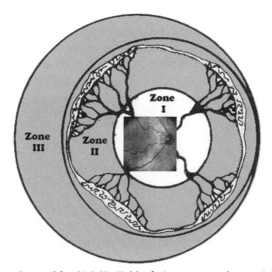

Fig. 9. Retinal zone imaged by SDOCT. Field of view range of retinal imaging with the portable handheld SDOCT unit. This system provides high-magnification imaging within zone I and can only infrequently capture images at the anterior border of zone I/posterior border of zone II. (*From* Lee AC, Maldonado RS, Sarin N, et al. Macular features from spectral-domain optical coherence tomography as an adjunct to indirect ophthalmoscopy in retinopathy of prematurity. Retina 2011;31(8):1470–82; with permission.)

NEW OCT IMAGING MODALITIES
Color Doppler OCT

Color Doppler OCT (CD-OCT) is a functional extension of OCT. By detecting the frequency shift of backscattered light, CD-OCT has been shown to be useful in measuring blood flow velocities and vascular perfusion. CD-OCT can provide qualitative and quantitative blood flow velocity assessments, although it is limited in clinical use because of imprecise information on the angle of the blood vessel relative to the scanning beam, which can limit precision of the data. In a laboratory experiment of fluid flow in capillary tubes, Hendargo and colleagues[25] showed the color representation of flow. Flow appears in the OCT image as a uniform colored circle (**Fig. 10**). As flow velocity increases, colored rings appear. The number of rings is directly proportional to the flow velocity. This phenomenon is called phase wrapping. When flow velocity exceeds the limit of phase wrapping detection, the Doppler signal disappears and the washout phenomenon occurs. There are no publications using Doppler in children for evaluation of retinal disease.

Enhanced Depth Imaging

Enhanced depth imaging (EDI) enables deeper structures such as the choroid to be better evaluated. This situation is important, because the choroid provides the oxygenation and support for the photoreceptors. Choroidal thickness has recently been linked in the pathophysiology of several retinal diseases, such as central serous retinopathy and macular degeneration. SDOCT devices decrease resolution with increasing displacement from the zero delay. By displacing the zero delay of the instrument to image deeper layers, the focused portion of the illumination is at the level of the choroid and inner sclera (**Fig. 11**).[26] There are no publications using this technique in children.

ROLE OF SDOCT IN ROP: BEYOND INDIRECT OPHTHALMOSCOPY

With SDOCT performed in neonates undergoing ROP screening, subclinical findings such as preretinal tissue (popcorn retinopathy), epiretinal membranes, cystoid macular changes, retinal layer schisis, precise localization of retinal detachment, vascular

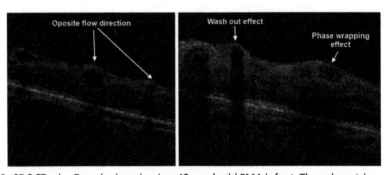

Fig. 10. SDOCT color Doppler imaging in a 42-week-old PMA infant. The volumetric scan was of 5 × 5 mm, 500 A-scans/B-scan, 40 B-scans and 5 Doppler samples (5 repeated A-scans at each single A-scan point). The B-scans shown were located in zone I across the temporal/superior vascular arcades. (*Left*) B-scan distal to the optic nerve. Red and blue represent vascular flow in opposite directions with respect to the OCT beam. (*Right*) B-scan more proximal to the optic nerve. Red and blue rings are produced by increased flow velocity. At higher flow velocities, the Doppler signal disappears, a phenomenon known as washout effect.

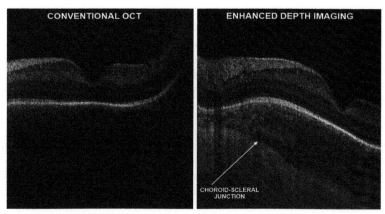

Fig. 11. Research SDOCT imaging with and without EDI in a 38-week-old PMA infant. With conventional SDOCT, the choroid may not always be well visualized, as shown in left panel. Furthermore, the choroid-scleral junction boundary is not clearly defined in the image. On the same infant, using EDI, which does not change the SDOCT signal directed into the eye, but modifying settings for the null point (*right*), the choroid features could be better appreciated and the choroid-scleral junction well defined without losing resolution of the retinal layers.

changes representative of plus disease, and cellular and subcellular changes related to ROP can be identified. These findings have been described in patients with aggressive posterior ROP[27] and patients with different degrees of ROP.[18,28]

For instance, in a study in 228 imaging sessions from 38 neonates undergoing ROP screening, Lee and colleagues[28] compared findings from conventional indirect ophthalmoscopy with vitreoretinal disease detected by SDOCT. These investigators found that SDOCT was better in detecting retinal cystoid structures in 39% of imaging sessions and epiretinal membranes in 32% and that most of these distorted foveal architecture. These 2 features were not visualized by indirect ophthalmoscopy in any of the infants. In contrast to ophthalmoscopic examination, SDOCT was not able to give information regarding ROP stage, zone, or vascular abnormality such as plus or preplus.

In ROP, functional outcomes are not always related to retinal structural outcomes, although there is a good correlation.[29] For example, in 606 eyes from the Early Treatment for Retinopathy of Prematurity Study (ETROP) study, Wallace and colleagues reported that 92 eyes (15.2%) had discordant outcomes: 86 eyes had unfavorable functional and favorable structural outcomes and 6 eyes had favorable functional and unfavorable structural outcomes. No OCT was available in that study, and thus the investigators could not rule out subclinical macular abnormalities. In the following sections, each ROP feature detectable with SDOCT is discussed.

Preretinal Tissue

Extraretinal isolated small masses of tissue lying over the retina can be visualized with SDOCT. We believe that these masses represent the fibrovascular isolated masses that have been described in the International Classification of ROP as isolated tissue that is not enough to meet criteria of stage 3 ROP. Traditionally, these masses have been known as popcorn retinopathy, located posterior to the ridge. OCT is an excellent methodology to evaluate preretinal tissue within zone I. Chavala and colleagues[27] described preretinal tissue in aggressive posterior ROP close to the optic nerve (**Fig. 12**). This tissue was visualized as thick rounded masses, causing intermittent shadows on OCT, which revealed the fibrovascular nature of the tissue. The capability of SDOCT to monitor preretinal tissue at early stages of the disease may play an important role in disease monitoring; for example, Wallace and colleagues[30] found that the presence of popcorn increases the risk of an eye with zone II stage 2 developing plus disease, stage 3, and requiring laser treatment.

Epiretinal Membranes

Epiretinal membranes are uncommon in children. They are formed by glial cells, retinal pigment epithelium cells, macrophages, vascular endothelial cells, fibrocytes, and collagen cells. The incidence in patients younger than 19 years is 1 in 20,896 and they are mostly related to trauma, idiopathic disease, and uveitis.[31] Thick epiretinal membranes have also been reported in stage 5 ROP in samples taken during vitrectomy.[32]

In the neonatal intensive care unit (NICU), epiretinal membranes are frequent, but these are seen generally as a thin hyperreflective line separated from the retinal surface (**Fig. 13**). For instance, Lee and colleagues[28] detected epiretinal membranes in 74 of 236 imaging sessions (32%) from 38 neonates ages 37.5 ± 4.8 weeks PMA. None of these epiretinal membranes was detected by ophthalmoscopy. One-third of the epiretinal membranes detected in the study produced foveal contour deformation.

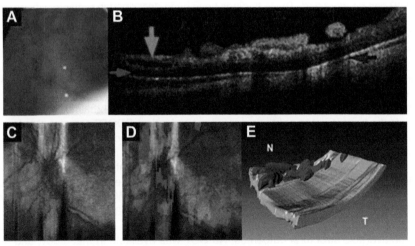

Fig. 12. Preretinal fibrovascular tissue in aggressive posterior ROP. Images obtained from the left eye of a 23-week-old born infant imaged at 37 weeks PMA. (*A*) Video-indirect image of the optic nerve and posterior pole of the retina without evidence of preretinal structures. (*B*) SDOCT B-scan showing preretinal tissue (*blue arrows*), retinal schisis (*green arrow*), subretinal fluid (*red arrow*), and denote shadowing artifact from preretinal structures (*purple arrow*). (*C*) Retinal image of optic nerve and posterior pole. (*D*) Same retinal image in (*C*) with preretinal tissue localized (*red areas* in *D*) surrounding and overlying optic nerve. (*E*) Three-dimensional SDOCT image reconstruction depicts preretinal structures in the posterior pole consistent with preretinal fibrovascular tissue. (*Modified from* Chavala SH, Farsiu S, Maldonado R, et al. Insights into advanced retinopathy of prematurity using handheld spectral domain optical coherence tomography imaging. Ophthalmology 2009;116:2450; with permission.)

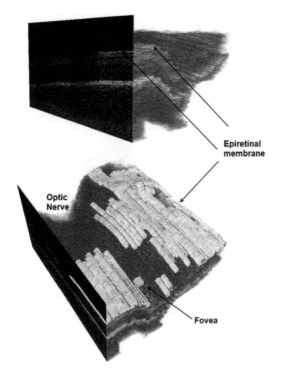

Fig. 13. Epiretinal membrane (ERM) in a 37-week-old PMA infant. Epiretinal membranes are frequent in infants with ROP but appear as a very thin hyperreflective layer separated from the retina (*top*) in contrast to thicker membranes seen in macular pucker. The lower figure aids in localization of the ERM, which is parafoveal and away from the optic nerve.

Macular Edema of Prematurity

A new insight into the pathophysiology of ROP is the finding of cystoid macular edema (CME) by SDOCT in premature infants throughout the prenatal period. With the benefit of SDSOCT imaging, it is shown that macular edema is a frequent finding in premature infants during their first months of life. Prominent cystoid hyporeflective spaces are located exclusively at the level of the inner nuclear layer in premature infant eyes (**Fig. 14**) and appear similar to cystoid spaces detected in some cases of diabetic macular edema or postcataract surgery.[9,17,28,33]

Because of the high frequency of this finding, plus the similar phenotype to macular edema seen in adult retinal diseases, this finding has been named macular edema of prematurity (MEOP).

In a study performed on 31 patients imaged from 31 to 42 weeks PMA (median birth weight 825 g, median gestational age 26 weeks PMA, final ROP stage <2), researchers found MEOP in 58% of patients.[9] The same researchers with a larger population group but considering imaging sessions 31 to 36 weeks PMA (median birth weight 760 g, median gestation age 26 weeks PMA, ROP stage 0–3) found CME in 50% of patients.[33] In both studies, CME was found in patients independently of ROP stage. Another study performed in 74 older and larger Asian-Indian neonates (average mean birth weight 1282 g, average gestational age 31 weeks PMA, ROP stages 0–2) found CME in 16% of patients, all of them with ROP stage 2, and found no CME in patients with stage 0 or 1 (**Table 4**).[17]

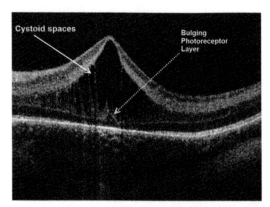

Cystoid spaces

Bulging
Photoreceptor
Layer

Fig. 14. Macular edema of prematurity. SDOCT cross-sectional image at the foveal center in a 38-week-old PMA infant. Prominent cystoid spaces located exclusively at the inner nuclear layer are characteristic of MEOP. Frequently, these spaces are vertically elongated and deform the fovea. Note the photoreceptor layer central dome, which is not expected at this age of development.

The studies mentioned earlier showed that MEOP is a transient event but the duration of edema is not well characterized. MEOP has been detected as early as 31 weeks PMA and resolved on its own. Vinekar and colleagues[17] showed CME resolution in 100% of patients. Maldonado and colleagues[33] reported resolution of CME as early as 36 weeks PMA, and the oldest age at which CME persisted was 43 weeks PMA. MEOP seems to be bilateral in most cases.

MEOP has different phenotypes and severity. Maldonado and colleagues[33] presented a morphologic classification of MEOP according to number, shape, location of cystoid structures, foveal pit morphology, and photoreceptor involvement (**Fig. 15**). Vinekar and colleagues[17] divided MEOP in 2 patterns: 1 with a dome-shaped fovea and 1 with preservation of foveal morphology. Both studies reported the bulging fovea with vertical elongated cysts to be the most prevalent.

Using robust image segmentation techniques, we have been able to provide a quantitative assessment of MEOP. Central foveal thickness (CFT) was found to be similar between both eyes of all patients, confirming the bilateral nature of this finding. The severity of MEOP, represented by CFT measurements, varied from 113 to 449 μm. This measure of CME severity in SDOCT imaging before 36 weeks PMA was found to be associated with final ROP disease stage and need for laser treatment (see **Table 5; Fig. 16**).[33] The bulge of the fovea was also objectively recorded in these infants using the ratio of foveal thickness/parafoveal thickness (1000 μm from foveal center) (foveal/parafoveal ratio) and found to be associated with final ROP disease stage and need for laser treatment.[33]

Now that the occurrence of MEOP in ROP is known, further research is needed to clarify questions about this event. Although MEOP is frequent and transient in premature infant eyes before term, it is still unclear if MEOP is a pathologic event or a transient local reaction during the first months of life in prematurely born neonates. In this regards, it is known that CME does not occur in healthy full-term neonates; Cabrera and colleagues[34] in a prospective observational study of 39 healthy full-term neonates did not find CME. In that study, 15% of neonates had subfoveal fluid similar to central serous retinopathy, which is a different event compared with CME. In premature infants, systemic factors such as gestational weight, birth weight, gender, race, surgery

Table 4 SDOCT studies in premature neonates undergoing ROP screening	Maldonado et al[33]	Vinekar et al[17]
Study Patient Characteristics		
Number of patients	42	74
Body weight (g)	760 (488–1032)	1282
Gestational age (wk PMA)	26 (25–27)	31 (30–33)
ROP stage	0–3	0–2
Plus	5	NR
Laser	12	0
Race		
White	17 (40.5)	0
African American	22 (52.4)	0
Asian	0	0
Hispanic	3 (7.1)	0
Indian	0	74 (100)
Age at Imaging (wk)		
Earliest imaging	30	35
Latest follow-up	43	52
MEOP, n (%)		
CME	21 (50)	12 (16)[a]
CFT	166 (91–449)	206 (108–304)
CME Characteristics		
Bilateral CME	21	NR
Bulging fovea	13 (62)	11 (47)
CME Resolution		
CME earliest resolution	36	NE
CME latest resolution	43	52

Abbreviations: CME, cystoid macular edema; NR, not reported.
[a] 23 eyes from a total of 146 eyes with ROP stages 0–2.

for Patent ductus arteriosus (PDA), sepsis, surgery for necrotizing enterocolitis (NEC), intraventricular hemorrhage, periventricular leukomalacia, bronchopulmonary dysplasia, and hydrocephalus have been evaluated and found not to be associated with the presence of MEOP.

There are some elements to support a possible pathologic role of MEOP. Number 1 is the fact that macular edema does not occur in all prematurely born neonates. Number 2 is the fact that it is exclusive to prematurely born neonates and not to healthy full-term neonates. Number 3 is the association found between MEOP severity and ROP outcome. Number 4 is the increased foveal thickness and abnormal foveal maturation found in older children with a history of ROP. Number 5 is the higher prevalence and severity of macular edema in infants of lower gestational age and lower birth weight.

If MEOP is a pathologic event, factors such as timing, duration, and severity of MEOP may be crucial in determining if foveal development and specifically photoreceptor development are affected. Visual function testing is needed to determine if MEOP has an adverse effect on normal foveal development or future visual acuity.

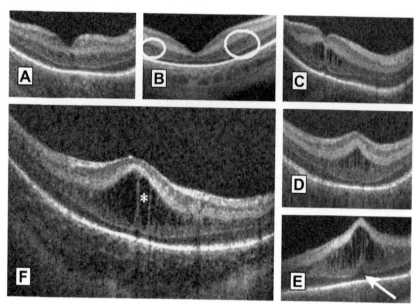

Fig. 15. Morphologic characteristics and phenotypes of MEOP in 42 prematurely born infants ages 31 to 37 weeks PMA. Three CME phenotypes were observed in the patients: (A) single central; (B) Parafoveal (when cystoid structures were grouped around the foveal center as shown within the white encircled areas), and (C) multiple elongated cystoid structures when the parafoveal and central fovea contained cystoid structures. For the multiple elongated CME phenotype, severity was scored as mild (C) if the foveal pit was present; moderate (D) if the fovea was bulging but Photoreceptor layer (PRL) was not affected and severe (E) when the fovea and PRL had a bulging shape (white arrow). (F) Magnified SDOCT scan to show morphologic characteristics found in severe CME. White asterisk is located within a cystoid space. (From Maldonado RS, O'Connell R, Ascher SB, et al. Spectral-domain optical coherence tomographic assessment of severity of cystoid macular edema in retinopathy of prematurity. Arch Ophthalmol 2012;130(5):572; with permission.)

Peripheral Retina, Retinoschisis, and Retinal Detachments: 4A Versus 4B

As discussed earlier, OCT is restricted to imaging the posterior pole. In a single volumetric scan, SDOCT can cover zone I ROP. If the handheld probe is tilted, the posterior zone II could be imaged. **Fig. 17** presents an example of stage 3 ROP obtained by tilting the probe toward the periphery. Muni and colleagues[18] also reported an image of stage 3 in a patient with ROP in zone I.

The determination of macular or foveal involvement in ROP retinal detachment is important in decision making and in predicting visual outcomes, and SDOCT imaging may be useful in making this determination. Not all eyes with 4A retinal detachment have a good functional outcome. Prener and colleagues[35] reported vision worse than 20/80 in 30% of cases undergoing pars-plana vitrectomy (PPV) for 4A detachment. Joshi and colleagues[15] showed the usefulness of OCT in determining foveal architecture abnormalities before surgery, which could explain why some patients did not do well despite a successfully attached retina. With SDOCT, the area detached can be mapped out and it can be distinguished with certainty if the fovea is involved or not, as shown in **Fig. 18**.

Table 5
Association of cystoid macular edema severity markers to ROP outcome found in 42 neonates imaged before 37 weeks PMA

Retinal Measurement	Progression to Laser Treatment in Study Eye			Vascular Outcome in Study Eye — Median (Range)			P Value	
	No (n = 30)	Yes (n = 12)	P Value	No Plus (n = 25)	Preplus (n = 6)	Plus (n = 11) No Plus	Plus vs No Plus	Preplus vs No Plus
CFT (μm)	145 (91–370)	236 (98–449)	.03	140 (91–370)	182 (104–329)	231 (98–449)	.046	.62
IRL thickness (μm)	108 (58–328)	194 (68–384)	.02	106 (65–328)	130 (58–215)	194 (68–384)	.02	.74
INL thickness (μm)	65 (32–263)	102 (46–316)	.11	65 (39–263)	55 (32–160)	102 (46–316)	.14	.40
PRL thickness (μm)	33 (13–65)	42 (22–59)	.20	29 (13–65)	46 (36–55)	42 (22–59)	.10	.80
Foveal/parafoveal ratio	0.65 (0.40–1.51)	1.09 (0.48–1.46)	.02	0.64 (0.40–1.36)	0.80 (0.43–1.51)	0.96 (0.48–1.46)	.03	.50

Abbreviations: CFT, central foveal thickness; CME, cystoid macular edema; FP, foveal-to-parafoveal; INL, inner nuclear layer; IRL, inner retinal layer; PRL, photoreceptor layer.

From Maldonado RS, O'Connell R, Ascher SB, et al. Spectral-domain optical coherence tomographic assessment of severity of cystoid macular edema in retinopathy of prematurity. Arch Ophthalmol 2012;130(5):569–78; with permission.

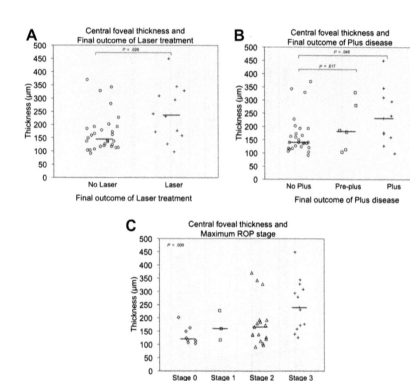

Fig. 16. CFT data distribution in premature infants imaged before 37 weeks PMA by final ROP outcome. The median CFT was significantly greater in the laser group than in the non-laser group (*A*), in the plus disease group than in the normal vasculature group (*B*), and in maximum stage 3 group than in patients with stages 0, 1, or 2 (*C*). (*From* Maldonado RS, O'Connell R, Ascher SB, et al. Spectral-domain optical coherence tomographic assessment of severity of cystoid macular edema in retinopathy of prematurity. Arch Ophthalmol 2012;130(5):573; with permission.)

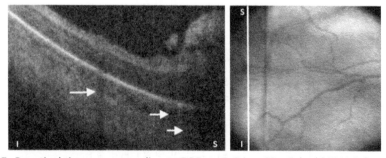

Fig. 17. Preretinal tissue corresponding to ROP stage 3 in a 32-week-old PMA infant. (*Left*) SDOCT B-scan of the periphery of zone I. The ridge and likely neovascularization appear as an elevated preretinal mass separated from the retina in some segments. These preretinal tissue cast shadows (*short white arrows*) because of its vascular component similar to the shadowing from retinal vessels (*longer white arrow*). (*Right*) Corresponding retinal image showing the location of the B-scan from left panel (*white line*).

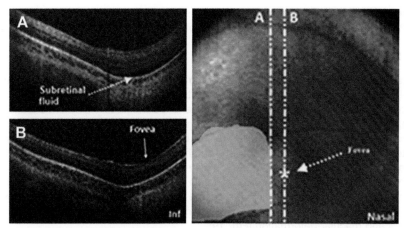

Fig. 18. SDOCT value in determination of foveal involvement in cases of retinal detachment. SDOCT imaging session performed in an infant diagnosed with retinal detachment caused by ROP. A 6 × 6 volumetric SDOCT scan of 80 B-scans was captured. Subretinal fluid was detected (*A*) and confirmed the retinal detachment. The fovea had no subretinal fluid present (*B*). Subretinal fluid was traced over the retinal image for estimation of retinal detachment size and localization.

Plus Disease

Plus disease is the most important clinical marker in ROP screening, essentially because it is the primary indication for laser treatment. The revised International Classification of ROP[36] defined a minor degree of vascular dilation and tortuosity named preplus, which has been shown to be predictive of progression to severe ROP requiring laser. Despite the clinical importance of these markers, there is disagreement among expert ROP examiners concerning plus and preplus.[37] Current research is aimed toward a more objective quantification of vascular dilation and tortuosity with computer software.

OCT can provide further insight in to vascular disease by showing the anatomic changes occurring in plus disease. For example, with OCT and three-dimensional reconstruction of OCT datasets, vessel tortuosity can be observed to occur in not only 2 dimensions but also in the third dimension across the depth of the retina. Furthermore, OCT characteristics are noted in the cross-sectional images that occur in plus disease such as vessel dilation and washout phenomenon, with Doppler imaging representing increased blood flow.

ROP, Choroid, and Photoreceptor Development

ROP affects the normal development of the human fovea. Studies performed in older children with a history of ROP have shown significantly higher CFT compared with controls.[38–40] Although it is commonly agreed that normal foveal development may be affected by ROP, until now it was not possible to assess when the insult affected the fovea. For the first time in history, we are able to observe, track, and quantify the in vivo development of the human fovea.[9] Maldonado and colleagues reported on foveal development from 31 weeks PMA up to adulthood, describing, with segmentation techniques, the centrifugal migration of retinal layer thickness and centripetal growth of photoreceptors. Furthermore, SDOCT studies performed during the period of foveal development were validated by comparing OCT images with histologic samples.[10,41] Choroid is another ocular element that might be affected or abnormal in ROP, and its relation to photoreceptor development is under evaluation.

DIFFERENT CLINICAL SCENARIOS

Portable SDOCT has the capability to accommodate a range of infant and child imaging. In this article, the application of SDOCT in the NICU is presented, which is perhaps the most challenging application, but other scenarios should also be mentioned, such as applications in clinic to imaging older infants with a history of ROP, or those who present with possible retinal disorder or unexplained decrease in vision with nystagmus, albinism, a history of trauma, or other optic nerve and retinal diseases. Between ages 6 months and 3 to 4 years, it may be difficult to approach the face of the young child for SDOCT imaging. SDOCT has been used during examinations under anesthesia and intraoperatively to differentiate retinal detachments involving the fovea and in older children with a history of ROP and to identify extent of epiretinal membranes and macular deformation (**Fig. 19**).

MAKING SENSE OF DATA
Segmentation Techniques

Robust segmentation techniques have been developed for studying adult retinal diseases. A customized segmentation technique was developed by Chiu and

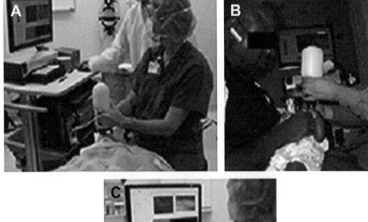

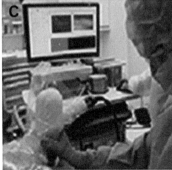

Fig. 19. Application of portable SDOCT in different clinical scenarios. In addition to the application of SDOCT in the NICU for infants undergoing ROP screening, portable SDOCT technology has been used, and published data have contributed to understanding of diverse retinal disease in infants and children undergoing examination under anesthesia (*A*), in the ophthalmologic pediatric clinic (*B*), and intraoperatively (*C*).

colleagues[42] to segment pediatric scans, which differ from adult scans in the number of layers at the foveal center (**Fig. 20**). This approach provides a more precise assessment of diseases and is semiautomatic.

Three-Dimensional Volume Rendering and Retinal Thickness Maps

Our laboratory has used computer software such as ImageJ (National Institutes of Health, Bethesda, MD, USA), MatLab (MathWorks, Natick, MA, USA), AVIZO (VSG Group, Burlington, MA, USA), and custom software to create three-dimensional data sets to map structures, shapes, and abnormalities. As shown in **Fig. 21**, retinal vessels, subretinal fluid, and preretinal tissue, among other features, can be localized to provide additional spatial information for understanding pathologic events and the foveal extent of abnormalities.

THE FUTURE

Combining current SDOCT system capabilities with a proper imaging methodology has proved the usefulness of OCT in providing novel information for the infant retina. This achievement is being translated into better understanding of structures, developmental mechanisms, and disease in ROP and other retinal diseases. Portable SDOCT takes us beyond the classic view of the retina and retinal vasculature. The information gathered by this imaging technology on the retina, choroid, and vessels may bring new insights in the pathophysiology of ROP.

Hardware modifications could enhance the usefulness of this imaging technology. For example, an increased SDOCT field of view may be of great use for evaluation of peripheral zones of ROP and extramacular retinal disease in infants. This modality will be useful in evaluating the avascular area and the vascular-avascular junction in ROP. Faster scanning could also be achieved with swept-source systems,[43] which can perform ultrahigh-speed imaging at more than 300,000 A-scans per second (see **Table 1**). This development could allow easier scan acquisition in restless babies or patients with nystagmus and would allow better Doppler imaging by reducing the scanning time required. Additional longitudinal studies relating the developmental and anomalous microanatomy to visual function outcomes are imperative to interpret infant anatomic OCT findings.

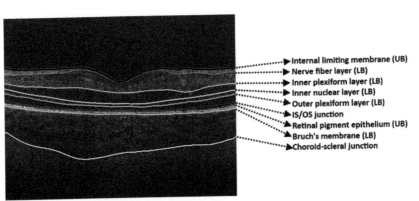

Internal limiting membrane (UB)
Nerve fiber layer (LB)
Inner plexiform layer (LB)
Inner nuclear layer (LB)
Outer plexiform layer (LB)
IS/OS junction
Retinal pigment epithelium (UB)
Bruch's membrane (LB)
Choroid-scleral junction

Fig. 20. Retinal layer segmentation on pediatric scans. Retinal layer boundaries segmented by DOCTRAP software. Nine retinal boundaries are detected and from these, retinal layer thicknesses can be calculated automatically.

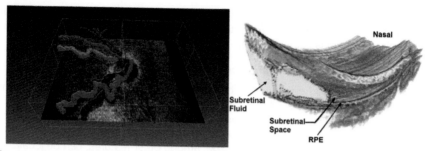

Fig. 21. Three-dimensional reconstruction from SDOCT scans captured in infants. Retinal vessels segmented (*left*) show tortuosity and help in distinguishing arterioles from venules. Subretinal fluid, retinal elevation, and retinal contour visualized in 3 dimensions using manual segmentation of subretinal fluid.

It is hoped that identifying early in the development of ROP eyes at greatest risk for lower visual acuity or other poor outcomes will allow for better and potentially new therapies for the disease. Furthermore, SDOCT may provide novel measurable end points for future treatments. It is an exciting present and a promising future for understanding mechanisms leading to different outcomes from ROP.

REFERENCES

1. Huang D, Swanson EA, Lin CP, et al. Optical coherence tomography. Science 1991;22:254.
2. Wojtkowski M, Leitgeb R, Kowalczyk A, et al. In vivo human retinal imaging by Fourier domain optical coherence tomography. J Biomed Opt 2002;7(3):457–63.
3. Yaqoob Z, Wu J, Yang C. Spectral domain optical coherence tomography: a better OCT imaging strategy. Biotechniques 2005;39(Suppl 6):S6–13.
4. Liu B, Brezinski ME. Theoretical and practical considerations on detection performance of time domain, Fourier domain, and swept source optical coherence tomography. J Biomed Opt 2012;12(4):044007.
5. Potsaid B, Baumann B, Huang D, et al. Ultrahigh speed 1050nm swept source/ Fourier domain OCT retinal and anterior segment imaging at 100,000 to 400,000 axial scans per second. Opt Express 2011;18(19):20029–48.
6. Fercher AF. Optical coherence tomography–development, principles, applications. Z Med Phys 2010;20(4):251–76.
7. Martin DF, Maguire MG, Fine SL, et al. Ranibizumab and bevacizumab for treatment of neovascular age-related macular degeneration: two-year results. Ophthalmology 2012;119(7):1388–98.
8. DeCroos FC, Toth CA, Stinnett SS, et al. Optical coherence tomography grading reproducibility during the comparison of age-related macular degeneration treatments trials. Ophthalmology 2012;119(12):2549–57.
9. Maldonado RS, O'Connell RV, Sarin N, et al. Dynamics of human foveal development after premature birth. Ophthalmology 2011;118(12):2315–25.
10. Vajzovic L, Hendrickson AE, O'Connell RV, et al. Maturation of the human fovea: correlation of spectral-domain optical coherence tomography findings with histology. Am J Ophthalmol 2012;154(5):779–789.e2.
11. Stopa M, Bower BA, Davies E, et al. Correlation of pathologic features in spectral domain optical coherence tomography with conventional retinal studies. Retina 2008;28(2):298–308.

12. World Health Organization. Vision for Children. A Global Overview of Blindness, Childhood and VISION 2020 The Right to Sight. London, UK; 2010.

13. Foster A. Childhood blindness. Eye (Lond) 1988;2(Suppl):S27–36.

14. Vinekar A, Sivakumar M, Shetty R, et al. A novel technique using spectral-domain optical coherence tomography (Spectralis, SD-OCT+HRA) to image supine non-anaesthetized infants: utility demonstrated in aggressive posterior retinopathy of prematurity. Eye (Lond) 2010;24(2):379–82.

15. Joshi MM, Trese MT, Capone A. Optical coherence tomography findings in stage 4A retinopathy of prematurity: a theory for visual variability. Ophthalmology 2006; 113(4):657–60.

16. Giordano VE, Hernandez-Vargas JA, Schoonewolff F. Comparison of optical coherence tomography macular findings in 5 year old patients with a history of pre-threshold or threshold retinopathy of prematurity treated with intravitreal bevacizumab as monotherapy, in ARVO meeting, Fort Lauderdale, FL, 2012.

17. Vinekar A, Avadhani K, Sivakumar M, et al. Understanding clinically unde-tected macular changes in early retinopathy of prematurity on spectral do-main optical coherence tomography. Invest Ophthalmol Vis Sci 2011;52(8): 5183–8.

18. Muni RH, Kohly RP, Charonis AC, et al. Retinoschisis detected with handheld spectral-domain optical coherence tomography in neonates with advanced retinopathy of prematurity. Arch Ophthalmol 2010;128(1):57–62.

19. Mactier H, Maroo S, Bradnam M, et al. Ocular biometry in preterm infants: impli-cations for estimation of retinal illuminance. Invest Ophthalmol Vis Sci 2008;49(1): 453–7.

20. Gordon RA, Donzis PB. Refractive development of the human eye. Arch Ophthal-mol 1985;103(6):785–9.

21. Cook A, White S, Batterbury M, et al. Ocular growth and refractive error develop-ment in premature infants with or without retinopathy of prematurity. Invest Ophthalmol Vis Sci 2008;49(12):5199–207.

22. Fledelius HC, Fledelius C. Eye size in threshold retinopathy of prematurity, based on a Danish preterm infant series: early axial eye growth, pre- and postnatal aspects. Invest Ophthalmol Vis Sci 2012;53(7):4177–84.

23. Lotmar W. A theoretical model for the eye of new-born infants. Albrecht Von Graefes Arch Klin Exp Ophthalmol 1976;198(2):179–85.

24. Maldonado RS, Izatt JA, Sarin N, et al. Optimizing hand-held spectral domain optical coherence tomography imaging for neonates, infants, and children. Invest Ophthalmol Vis Sci 2010;51(5):2678–85.

25. Hendargo HC, McNabb RP, Dhalla AH, et al. Doppler velocity detection limita-tions in spectrometer-based versus swept-source optical coherence tomography. Biomed Opt Express 2011;2(8):2175–88.

26. Spaide RF, Koizumi H, Pozzoni MC, et al. Enhanced depth imaging spectral-domain optical coherence tomography. Am J Ophthalmol 2008;146(4):496–500.

27. Chavala SH, Farsiu S, Maldonado R, et al. Insights into advanced retinopathy of prematurity using handheld spectral domain optical coherence tomography imaging. Ophthalmology 2009;116(12):2448–56.

28. Lee AC, Maldonado RS, Sarin N, et al. Macular features from spectral-domain optical coherence tomography as an adjunct to indirect ophthalmoscopy in reti-nopathy of prematurity. Retina 2011;31(8):1470–82.

29. Wallace DK, Bremer DL, Good WV, et al. Correlation of recognition visual acuity with posterior retinal structure in advanced retinopathy of prematurity. Arch Oph-thalmol 2012;130(12):1512–6.

30. Wallace DK, Kylstra JA, Greenman DB, et al. Significance of isolated neovascular tufts ('popcorn') in retinopathy of prematurity. J AAPOS 1998;2(1):52–6.
31. Khaja HA, McCannel CA, Diehl NN, et al. Incidence and clinical characteristics of epiretinal membranes in children. Arch Ophthalmol 2008;126(5):632–6.
32. Fei P, Zhao PQ, Chen RJ, et al. Histopathological study of epiretinal membranes in retinopathy of prematurity. Zhonghua Yan Ke Za Zhi 2008;44(7):629–33 [in Chinese].
33. Maldonado RS, O'Connell R, Ascher SB, et al. Spectral-domain optical coherence tomographic assessment of severity of cystoid macular edema in retinopathy of prematurity. Arch Ophthalmol 2012;130(5):569–78.
34. Cabrera MT, Maldonado RS, Toth CA, et al. Subfoveal fluid in healthy full-term newborns observed by handheld spectral-domain optical coherence tomography. Am J Ophthalmol 2012;153(1):167–75.
35. Prenner JL, Capone A, Trese MT. Visual outcomes after lens-sparing vitrectomy for stage 4A retinopathy of prematurity. Ophthalmology 2004;111(12):2271–3.
36. International Committee for the Classification of Retinopathy of Prematurity. The International Classification of Retinopathy of Prematurity revisited. Arch Ophthalmol 2005;123(7):991–9.
37. Wallace DK, Quinn GE, Freedman SF, et al. Agreement among pediatric ophthalmologists in diagnosing plus and pre-plus disease in retinopathy of prematurity. J AAPOS 2008;12(4):352–6.
38. Children F, Ecsedy M, Szamosi A, et al. A comparison of macular structure imaged by optical coherence tomography in preterm and full-term children. Invest Ophthalmol Vis Sci 2007;48(11):5207–11.
39. Park KA, Oh SY. Analysis of spectral-domain optical coherence tomography in preterm children: retinal layer thickness and choroidal thickness profiles. Invest Ophthalmol Vis Sci 2012;53(11):7201–7.
40. Recchia FM, Recchia CC. Foveal dysplasia evident by optical coherence tomography in patients with a history of retinopathy of prematurity. Retina 2006;27(9):1221–6.
41. Dubis AM, Costakos DM, Subramaniam CD, et al. Evaluation of normal human foveal development using optical coherence tomography and histologic examination. Arch Ophthalmol 2012;130(10):1291–300.
42. Chiu SJ, Li XT, Nicholas P, et al. Automatic segmentation of seven retinal layers in SDOCT images congruent with expert manual segmentation. Opt Express 2010;18(18):19413.
43. Drexler W, Fujimoto JG. State-of-the-art retinal optical coherence tomography. Prog Retin Eye Res 2008;27(1):45–88.

Current and Future Trends in Treatment of Severe Retinopathy of Prematurity

David K. Wallace, MD, MPH[a],*, Katherine Y. Wu, BS[a,b]

KEYWORDS

- Retinopathy of prematurity • Type 1 • Laser photocoagulation • Bevacizumab
- Clinical trials • Side effects

KEY POINTS

- Treatment for retinopathy of prematurity (ROP) is indicated when type 1 disease is present.
- The Early Treatment for Retinopathy of Prematurity (ETROP) clinical trial established that laser treatment of severe ROP has a high rate of visual and anatomic success.
- Recently, anti-vascular endothelial growth factor (VEGF) drugs, such as bevacizumab, have been used in lieu of or in addition to laser treatment.
- Results with bevacizumab are promising, but long-term outcomes and systemic side effects are unknown.
- Future studies are needed to determine whether anti-VEGF treatment is superior to laser and, if so, which drug and dose are safe and effective.

INTRODUCTION

The Early Treatment for Retinopathy of Prematurity (ETROP) study established the guidelines currently in use for optimal timing of laser treatment for severe retinopathy of prematurity (ROP).[1] The ETROP study concluded that ROP should be treated when type 1 ROP is present, which is defined as: (1) Zone I, any stage with plus disease, or (2) Zone I, stage 3 without plus disease, or (3) Zone 2, stage 2 or 3 with plus disease. Because Zone I, stage 3 ROP without plus disease is uncommon, most cases of type 1 ROP have plus disease. Treatment for disease less severe than type 1, including type 2 prethreshold ROP, is not indicated. Type 2 ROP is defined as Zone I, stage 1 or 2 without plus disease, or Zone II, stage 3 without plus disease. Eyes with type 2 ROP should not be treated, but instead should be observed for development of

Financial Disclosure: D.K. Wallace is a consultant for Genentech.
[a] Department of Ophthalmology and Pediatrics, Duke Eye Center, 2351 Erwin Road, Durham, NC 27710, USA; [b] Duke University School of Medicine, Durham, NC, USA
* Corresponding author.
E-mail address: david.wallace@duke.edu

type 1 ROP. In the ETROP study, the rate of unfavorable visual acuity at age 6 years for type 2 prethreshold eyes was 23.6% for eyes treated as high risk prethreshold and 19.4% for those managed conventionally ($P = .37$).[2] In addition, many eyes recover without treatment. Even among high-risk prethreshold eyes in the ETROP study, 52% regressed without treatment.[1]

LASER TREATMENT FOR SEVERE ROP

Laser photocoagulation is a time-tested, very successful treatment for severe ROP. Before the advent of laser treatment, cryotherapy was the first treatment shown to be effective for severe ROP. In the Cryotherapy for Retinopathy of Prematurity (CRYO-ROP) study, eyes of 291 infants with threshold ROP were randomized to cryotherapy or observation. After 12 months, the rate of unfavorable anatomic outcome (defined as a macular fold or detachment, a retrolental mass, or surgery for a retinal detachment) was 47% in the untreated eyes and 26% in the treated eyes.[3] Over time, laser replaced cryotherapy as the preferred method for treating peripheral avascular retina.

ETROP study investigators hypothesized that eyes treated earlier than threshold (ie, high-risk prethreshold) would have a better outcome. In this study, an unfavorable visual acuity outcome was defined as greater than 4 standard deviations from the mean for age by Teller Acuity Cards. The rates of unfavorable visual acuity at 9 months were 14.5% in eyes treated at high risk prethreshold, and 19.5% in conventionally managed eyes. Unfavorable retinal structure at 9 months was even better. Eyes treated at high risk prethreshold had an unfavorable visual acuity outcome rate of 9.1%, and those managed conventionally had a 15.6% unfavorable rate.[1] Six-year outcomes from the ETROP study confirmed that eyes with type 1 ROP benefited from treatment at high risk prethreshold. Twenty-five percent of those eyes had an unfavorable outcome (defined as visual acuity of 20/200 or worse) using Early Treatment Diabetic Retinopathy Study acuity.[2]

Laser treatment has several advantages. It has a very high success rate in terms of favorable visual outcome and avoiding retinal detachment. However, for many children, a favorable outcome does not mean normal vision.[4] There may be effects of ROP or its treatment on the developing macula that are not seen by indirect ophthalmoscopy. For example, spectral-domain optical coherence tomography has shown cystoid structures and epiretinal membranes that are not detectable by routine examination.[5] Laser treatment of ROP has been used successfully for many years, and the treatment itself has no systemic side effects. Sedation or intubation, sometimes required for treatment, may have systemic effects. Laser treatment does have some disadvantages. It is more time-consuming than is giving an intravitreal injection. It is more expensive than an injection of bevacizumab, which is the most commonly used anti–vascular endothelial growth factor (VEGF) treatment for ROP. There is a learning curve with delivery of effective laser treatment, and the necessary equipment and trained personnel are not available in all countries. Retreatment with laser is needed in approximately 10% of cases, but varies by practice, as some physicians deliver a higher number or intensity of laser spots during the initial treatment session. Prolonged laser treatment can cause upper back and neck pain for treating physicians. Possible ocular side effects of laser include cataracts, inflammation, hyphema, and phthisis.

ANTI-VEGF TREATMENT FOR SEVERE ROP

VEGF is important in the pathogenesis of ROP. Retinal ischemia causes excessive accumulation of VEGF, which results in the neovascularization that characterizes severe ROP.[6] As such, anti-VEGF drugs are a more direct approach than laser in blocking the effects of VEGF on the retina. Laser destroys peripheral avascular retina, which results in less VEGF production, but the effect is less rapid than with anti-VEGF treatment. Four anti-VEGF drugs are bevacizumab (Avastin), ranibizumab (Lucentis), pegaptanib (Macugen), and aflibercept (VEGF trap); of these, bevacizumab has been used the most in premature infants. An injection of bevacizumab is less time-consuming and less expensive than laser treatment. **Fig. 1** shows both eyes of a premature infant with type 1 ROP in Zone I, before bevacizumab injection and then 1 day after injection. Several case series have reported rapid resolution and high rates of success after bevacuzimab,[7–11] and there has been one randomized trial (BEAT-ROP study) suggesting that anti-VEGF treatment is superior to laser for severe ROP in Zone I.[12] **Table 1** summarizes results from studies published to date on the treatment of severe ROP with anti-VEGF injections.

BEAT-ROP STUDY

There has been one published randomized trial comparing bevacizumab with laser for severe ROP. The BEAT-ROP (Bevacizumab Eliminates the Angiogenic Threat of ROP) study randomized infants to receive laser or bevacizumab, 0.625 mg in 0.025 mL. All infants had Zone I or posterior Zone II, stage 3 ROP with plus disease. The primary outcome was "recurrence of neovascularization in 1 or 2 eyes requiring retreatment by 54 weeks postmenstrual age." The study found that 6 of 140 eyes (4%) receiving bevacizumab had recurrence of neovascularization, compared with 32 of 146 lasered eyes (22%, $P = .002$). For Zone I, there was a statistically significant difference in recurrence rate between groups ($P = .003$), and for Zone II, there was no difference

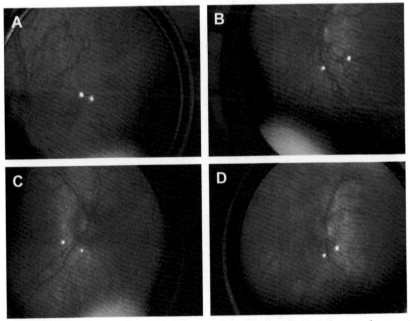

Fig. 1. Pre-injection of (*A*) Right eye of premature infant and (*B*) Left eye of premature infant. 1 day after intravitreal injection of 0.625 mg bevacizumab of (*C*) Right eye and (*D*) Left eye.

Table 1
Summary of results from studies published to date on treatment of severe ROP with anti-VEGF injections

Authors,[Ref.] Year	Study Design	No. of Patients	ROP Severity of Patients	Treatment	Outcome	Retreatment	Complications	Follow-up
Quiroz-Mercado et al,[9] 2008	Noncomparative, prospective, interventional case series	13 patients (18 eyes)	*Group I:* Stage 4a or 4b ROP that had no response to conventional treatment (3 patients, 4 eyes) *Group II:* Patients with threshold ROP and poor visualization of the retina (5 patients, 5 eyes) *Group III:* Patients with high-risk prethreshold or threshold ROP (5 patients, 9 eyes)	1 intravitreal injection of 1.25 mg bevacizumab as initial therapy	Neovascular regression in all patients	Not applicable	None	Mean follow-up of 6 mo after injection

Study	Design	Sample	Groups	Treatment	Outcomes	Additional Treatment	Complications	Follow-up
Roohipoor et al,[10] 2011	Interventional case series	10 patients (12 eyes)	*Group 1:* Threshold ROP that did not respond to laser or had complications after laser (8 eyes) *Group 2:* Aggressive Posterior ROP (APROP) with no prior treatment (4 eyes)	*Group 1:* 1 intravitreal injection of 0.625 mg bevacizumab after laser *Group 2:* 1 intravitreal injection of 0.625 mg bevacizumab as initial therapy	*Group 1:* All eyes had regression of neovascularization (NV), resorption of vitreous hemorrhage (VH), and disappearance of hyphema in first week *Group 2:* 1 patient had regression of ROP and complete peripheral vascularization; 1 patient had regression in plus disease, incomplete vascularization	*Group 1:* Not applicable *Group 2:* 1 patient required laser treatment 1.5 mo after bevacizumab	None	At least 1 y

(continued on next page)

Table 1
(continued)

Authors,[Ref.] Year	Study Design	No. of Patients	ROP Severity of Patients	Treatment	Outcome	Retreatment	Complications	Follow-up
Wu et al,[11] 2011	Multicenter, retrospective case series study	27 patients (49 eyes)	*Stage 3 ROP:* 23 patients (41 eyes, 9 of which are Zone 1 and 32 are Zone 2) *Stage 4A ROP:* 3 patients (6 eyes) *Stage 5 ROP:* 1 patient (2 eyes)	*Stage 3 ROP:* 36 eyes (88%) received 1 intravitreal injection of 0.625 mg bevacizumab as initial therapy 5 eyes (12%) received 0.625 mg bevacizumab as salvage therapy after no response to laser *Stage 4 and 5 ROP:* 0.625 mg Bevacizumab was used to reduce chance of bleeding during vitrectomy	*Stage 3 ROP:* 37 of 41 eyes (90%) regressed *Stage 4a ROP:* 2 eyes (33%) regressed without need for vitrectomy *Stage 5 ROP:* 2 eyes displayed decreased vascular tortuosity after treatment	*Stage 3 ROP:* 4 eyes (10%) required additional laser *Stage 4a ROP:* 4 eyes (67%) regressed after bevacizumab + vitrectomy *Stage 5:* 2 eyes had retina fail to reattach after multiple vitrectomy surgeries	Vitreous or preretinal hemorrhage in 4 eyes (8%). Eventually resolved in all eyes Transient vascular sheathing in inferior venous branch in 2 eyes (4%)	At least 6 mo following treatment

Mintz-Hittner et al,[12] 2011	Prospective, controlled, randomized, stratified, multicenter trial	143 patients (286 eyes)	Zone I or posterior Zone II stage 3+	1 intravitreal injection of 0.625 mg bevacizumab, bilaterally, as initial therapy OR Conventional laser therapy, bilaterally, as initial therapy	Bevacizumab group: *Recurrence of NV with Zone I disease in 4 of 62 eyes *Recurrence of NV with Zone II disease in 4 of 78 eyes Laser group: *Recurrence of NV with Zone 1 disease in 28 of 66 eyes ($P = .003$) *Recurrence of NV with Zone II disease in 10 of 80 eyes ($P = .27$)	Need for additional treatment was the primary outcome	1 case of corneal opacity, 3 cases of lens opacity with laser therapy	54 wk postmenstrual age
Hu et al,[14] 2012	Retrospective review	9 patients (17 eyes) Only patients that had recurrence of ROP after bevacizumab were included	Type 1 ROP	1 intravitreal injection of 0.625–0.75 mg bevacizumab	Initial regression of ROP 5 eyes progressed to retinal detachment (RD) (mean age of RD was 58.4 wk postmenstrual age, minimum = 49 wk, maximum = 69 wk)	Mean age at treatment-requiring recurrence was 49.3 wk postmenstrual age Retreatment consisted of repeated injections, and/or laser, and/or surgical repair	1 eye had cataract presumably associated with injection	56–104 wk

(continued on next page)

Table 1
(continued)

Authors,[Ref.] Year	Study Design	No. of Patients	ROP Severity of Patients	Treatment	Outcome	Retreatment	Complications	Follow-up
Wu et al,[18] 2013	Multicenter, retrospective case series	85 patients (162 eyes)	Type 1 ROP	1 intravitreal injection of 0.625 mg bevacizumab as initial therapy	143 eyes (88%) exhibited ROP regression	14 eyes (9%) required additional laser treatment 2 eyes (1%) required 1 additional injection	2 eyes (1%) had vitreous or preretinal hemorrhage 1 eye (1%) had cataract	Until full vascularization of retina was observed (average of 13.7 mo)
Nazari et al,[19] 2010	Prospective, interventional case series	8 patients (14 eyes)	Severe ROP associated with VH or retinal hemorrhage (RH) 8 eyes had VH and/or RH precluding laser 6 eyes had VH develop after laser	1 intravitreal injection of 0.625 mg bevacizumab as initial therapy	In all eyes, plus disease disappeared completely within 2 wk and VH and/or RH was absorbed at last follow-up	Not applicable	None	3 mo after injection

Harder et al,[20] 2011	Retrospective chart analysis	12 patients (23 eyes)	Threshold ROP	1 intravitreal injection of 0.375 mg bevacizumab as initial therapy	All eyes showed regression of plus disease within 2–6 d, decrease in pupillary rigidity, resolution of any tunica vasculosa lentis, if present before injection, and complete regression of retinal NV within 2–3 wk	Not applicable	None	Mean follow-up 30.4 wk
				1 eye of 1 infant received laser then 0.375 mg bevacizumab owing to progression of disease	The eye that received laser and then bevacizumab developed a retinal fold and macular ectopia			

(continued on next page)

Table 1
(continued)

Authors,[Ref.] Year	Study Design	No. of Patients	ROP Severity of Patients	Treatment	Outcome	Retreatment	Complications	Follow-up
Lee et al,[21] 2012	Retrospective review	3 patients (5 eyes) Patients were referred to tertiary care center for management of fibrous retinal traction band	Stage 3 ROP with plus	1 intravitreal injection of 0.75 mg bevacizumab as initial therapy (1 eye) 1 intravitreal injection of 0.75 mg bevacizumab + laser (4 eyes)	In all patients, initial regression of extraretinal fibrovascular proliferation and initial regression of plus disease In all patients, within 2.5–4 mo of initial ROP regression, atypical fibrous traction membrane developed Tractional RD in 3 of 5 eyes	Not applicable	None	19–31 mo after treatment (mean 23 mo)
Dorta and Kychenthal,[22] 2010	Noncomparative, consecutive case series	7 patients (12 eyes)	Type 1 ROP (9 eyes had Zone I, 3 had Zone II)	1 intravitreal injection of 0.625 mg bevacizumab as initial therapy	All eyes showed regression of disease	Not applicable	1 eye had an epiretinal hemorrhage due to injection procedure	Until vascularization reached Zone III
Salman,[23] 2010	Prospective, nonrandomized study	9 patients (18 eyes)	Stage 3, threshold, or plus disease in Zone I/II	1 intravitreal injection of 0.625 mg bevacizumab as initial therapy	12 eyes had reduced neovascular activity after 1 injection	4 eyes required 2 injections 2 eyes needed 3 injections	None	1 y

between groups ($P = .27$).[12] This study had several important limitations. The primary outcome of recurrent neovascularization depended on treatment decisions by unmasked investigators. In addition, this outcome is considerably less relevant than visual acuity or retinal structure. Second, the laser "failure rate" of 22% was much higher than that reported in other studies, such as the ETROP study. Third, no safety data were provided.

UNKNOWNS/POTENTIAL DISADVANTAGES OF ANTI-VEGF TREATMENT

Disadvantages of anti-VEGF treatment include the risk for endophthalmitis with intravitreal injection, unknown neural retinal effects, the possible effects of anti-VEGF on developing organs in the systemic circulation,[13] a possibly higher death rate,[12] and the need for extended follow-up in the outpatient setting because of late recurrence of severe ROP.[14]

Serum VEGF levels decrease significantly after intravitreal injection in infants with ROP. In one study, bevacizumab levels increased from 1 day to 1 week to 2 weeks after injection.[15] The effects on developing organs in the fragile premature infant are unknown. Some investigators have presented case series of infants treated with anti-VEGF drugs and have stated that "there have been no systemic side effects," but such a conclusion cannot be established without a randomized comparison group. In a cohort of premature infants, there is much comorbidity, including developmental delay and cerebral palsy. If, for example, an anti-VEGF drug adversely affects the brain, this can only be known by comparing the neurodevelopment of infants randomized to treatment with that in children without the study drug.

Late recurrence of ROP has been observed in some cases after bevacizumab injection.[14] It is unknown how often this occurs, how it should be treated, and how long these infants need to be closely followed after anti-VEGF injection. Additional clinical studies, including randomized trials, are needed to address many of these unanswered questions.

OUR CURRENT APPROACH

The current approach is based on the fact that laser has a high success rate, and the failure rate reflects the ETROP experience. Therefore, most babies with Zone I or Zone II ROP will undergo laser treatment. Bevacizumab also seems to have a high success rate. Which of the two treatments is better for infants with type 1 ROP has not yet been established. Data from the BEAT-ROP study showed a lower rate of recurrent neovascularization requiring retreatment with bevacizumab in comparison with laser.[12] However, there are different types of Zone I eyes. For example, there are Zone I eyes with a ridge that is close to or straddling the border of Zone 2. These eyes tend to act like Zone II eyes and usually respond well to laser treatment. On the other hand, there are eyes that resemble a postage stamp, which have a very small amount of vascularization and no visible macula and whose vessels do not extend far from the optic nerve. Bevacizumab is a particularly promising treatment for these types of eyes.

FUTURE DIRECTIONS

A large clinical trial comparing anti-VEGF treatment with laser is needed, with data on outcomes of visual acuity, retinal structure, and nerve development. Clinicians need to know how these treatments compare for short-term and long-term outcomes of (1) visual acuity by blinded examiners and (2) retinal structure, which would ideally be based on grading of the images by blinded experts. Moreover, data are needed to compare outcomes when the laser failure rate is similar to that shown by ETROP. In the BEAT-ROP study, the laser failure rate was much higher than that found by most investigators who treat severe ROP. A larger trial could include intensive monitoring for systemic side effects and information about rare events, such as death, that can only be gleaned from a large cohort.

Which Drug?

Which anti-VEGF drug is the best to use for ROP? When choosing which drug to use, factors to consider are efficacy, systemic effects, and cost. The amount of drug crossing the ocular-blood barrier is not just a function of molecular size, because there are receptors that can facilitate the transport of entire molecules of immunoglobulin G.[16] In adults, ranibizumab has a shorter half-life than bevacizumab in the systemic circulation.[17] Comparative data on pharmacokinetics and systemic side effects in premature infants are required.

Which Dose?

Once the best anti-VEGF drug is known, what is the best dose? Dosing studies can be done as part of the nonrandomized, phase 1 clinical trial. One strategy would be to start with an effective dose and then gradually reduce the dose, using preestablished criteria for success at each dose level.

Which Treatment Strategy?

There is a plethora of new information about anti-VEGF treatment, which must all be put together into an evidence-based treatment paradigm. Possible treatment paradigms include: (1) laser for all type 1 cases followed by anti-VEGF as salvage treatment if laser fails; (2) laser for most cases and then anti-VEGF for very posterior Zone 1, obstructed view for laser, or when laser is not available; (3) laser for some cases, anti-VEGF for all Zone 1 cases and Zone 2 cases with an obstructed view; or (4) anti-VEGF as the primary therapy for all cases. If anti-VEGF is used as primary therapy for all cases of type 1 ROP, it could be followed by laser in all cases, or it could be followed by additional treatment for cases with recurrent disease. Additional treatment might consist of laser photocoagulation or reinjection of anti-VEGF treatment. Regarding the best approach, uncontrolled observational data may suggest that anti-VEGF treatment is effective without causing significant systemic side effects, but only high-quality comparisons of different approaches will truly guide us. Although nonrandomized retrospective or prospective data can be helpful, randomized controlled trials are the gold standard for guiding future treatments.

Need for Additional Studies

There is a long way to go to before an evidence-based treatment paradigm for laser and anti-VEGF therapy is available. Even before we pursue large randomized trials we still need to know which drug, which dose, and which treatment strategies to compare. There are many opportunities for high-quality comparative studies to shape the future treatment of severe ROP.

REFERENCES

1. Early Treatment for Retinopathy of Prematurity Cooperative Group. Revised indications for the treatment of retinopathy of prematurity: results of the early treatment for retinopathy of prematurity randomized trial. Arch Ophthalmol 2003; 121:1684–94.

2. Early Treatment for Retinopathy of Prematurity Cooperative Group, Good WV, Hardy RJ, Dobson V, et al. Final visual acuity results in the early treatment for retinopathy of prematurity study. Arch Ophthalmol 2010;128:663–71.
3. Cryotherapy for Retinopathy of Prematurity Cooperative Group. Multicenter trial of cryotherapy for retinopathy of prematurity one-year outcome: structure and function. Arch Ophthalmol 1990;108(10):1408–16.
4. Wallace DK, Bremer DL, Good WV, et al. Correlation of recognition visual acuity with posterior retinal structure in advanced retinopathy of prematurity. Arch Ophthalmol 2012;13:1–5.
5. Lee AC, Maldonado RS, Sarin N, et al. Macular features from spectral-domain optical coherence tomography as an adjunct to indirect ophthalmoscopy in retinopathy of prematurity. Retina 2011;31:1470–82.
6. Smith LE. Through the eyes of a child: understanding retinopathy through ROP the Friedenwald lecture. Invest Ophthalmol Vis Sci 2008;49:5177–82.
7. Dani C, Frosini S, Fortunato P, et al. Intravitreal bevacizumab for retinopathy of prematurity as first line or rescue therapy with focal laser treatment. A case series. J Matern Fetal Neonatal Med 2012;25:2194–7.
8. Kusaka S, Shima C, Wada K, et al. Efficacy of intravitreal injection of bevacizumab for severe retinopathy of prematurity: a pilot study. Br J Ophthalmol 2008; 92:1450–5.
9. Quiroz-Mercado H, Martinez-Castellanos MA, Hernandez-Rojas ML, et al. Antiangiogenic therapy with intravitreal bevacizumab for retinopathy of prematurity [Erratum appears in Retina 2009;29(1):127]. Retina 2008;28(Suppl):S19–25.
10. Roohipoor R, Ghasemi H, Ghassemi F, et al. Intravitreal bevacizumab in retinopathy of prematurity: an interventional case series. Graefes Arch Clin Exp Ophthalmol 2011;249:1295–301.
11. Wu WC, Yeh PT, Chen SN, et al. Effects and complications of bevacizumab use in patients with retinopathy of prematurity: a multicenter study in Taiwan. Ophthalmology 2011;118:176–83.
12. Mintz-Hittner HA, Kennedy KA, Chuang AZ, BEAT-ROP Cooperative Group. Efficacy of intravitreal bevacizumab for stage 3 retinopathy of prematurity. N Engl J Med 2011;364:603–15.
13. Darlow BA, Ells AL, Gilbert CE, et al. Are we there yet? Bevacizumab therapy for retinopathy of prematurity. Arch Dis Child Fetal Neonatal Ed 2013;98(2): F170–4.
14. Hu J, Blair MP, Shapiro MJ, et al. Reactivation of retinopathy of prematurity after bevacizumab injection. Arch Ophthalmol 2012;130:1000–6.
15. Sato T, Wada K, Arahori H, et al. Serum concentrations of bevacizumab (Avastin) and vascular endothelial growth factor in infants with retinopathy of prematurity. Am J Ophthalmol 2012;153:327–33.
16. Kim H, Robinson SB, Csaky KG. FcRn receptor-mediated pharmacokinetics of therapeutic IgG in the eye. Mol Vis 2009;15:2803–12.
17. Tolentino M. Systemic and ocular safety of intravitreal anti-VEGF therapies for ocular neovascular disease. Surv Ophthalmol 2011;56:95–113.
18. Wu WC, Kuo HK, Yeh PT, et al. An updated study of the use of bevacizumab in the treatment of patients with prethreshold retinopathy of prematurity in Taiwan. Am J Ophthalmol 2013;155:150–8.
19. Nazari H, Modarres M, Parvaresh MM, et al. Intrvitreal bevacizumab in combination with laser therapy for the treatment of severe retinopathy of prematurity (ROP) associated with vitreous or retinal hemorrhage. Graefes Arch Clin Exp Ophthalmol 2010;248:1713–8.

20. Harder BC, von Baltz S, Jonas JB, et al. Intravitreal bevacizumab for retinopathy of prematurity. J Ocul Pharmacol Ther 2011;27:623–7.

21. Lee BJ, Kim JH, Heo H, et al. Delayed onset atypical vitreoretinal traction band formation after an intravitreal injection of bevacizumab in stage 3 retinopathy of prematurity. Eye (Lond) 2012;26:903–9.

22. Dorta P, Kychenthal A. Treatment of type 1 retinopathy of prematurity with intravitreal bevacizumab (Avastin). Retina 2010;30(Suppl 4):S24–31.

23. Salman AG. Intravitreal bevacizumab injection as a primary therapy for threshold disease (ROP) in Al Qassim region. J Clin Exp Ophthalmol 2010;1:113.

Outcome of Retinopathy of Prematurity

Gerd Holmström, MD, PhD*, Eva Larsson, MD, PhD*

KEYWORDS

- Retinopathy of prematurity • Prematurity • Outcome • Follow-up • Visual function

KEY POINTS

- The outcome of visual functions, such as visual acuity, visual fields, strabismus, contrast sensitivity, accommodation, and convergence, in prematurely born children is discussed.
- The anatomic outcome of retinopathy of prematurity and preterm birth, such as refraction, retinal anatomy, and morphology is discussed.
- The clinical follow-up of prematurely born children with and without retinopathy of prematurity is discussed.

Various ophthalmologic sequelae occur in prematurely born children, and the overall outcome of retinopathy of prematurity (ROP) has changed over time. The prevalence of visual and ophthalmologic problems varies with the standard of neonatal care and socioeconomic situation, as shown by Gilbert,[1] who reported a low risk of childhood blindness caused by ROP in rich countries and a high risk in middle-income countries, whereas it rarely existed in poor countries. In developed countries, improved neonatal care, improved screening for ROP, and more efficient treatment have reduced the prevalence of sequelae attributable to ROP, which was recently shown in a study from the Netherlands comparing results over the last 30 years.[2]

Several long-term ophthalmologic studies of the outcome of preterm birth and ROP have been published, although different methodologies and inclusion criteria may have led to different results. Most of the studies are hospital-based, and only a few of the studies that extend up to school age or adolescence, in which children were also screened for ROP, are population based (**Table 1**). Reports of sequelae in the adult population are mostly follow-up studies of eyes with ROP before treatment was introduced.[3,4] The long-term outcome of treated ROP per se has been reported in selected studies, such as the American Cryotherapy for Retinopathy of Prematurity

No financial disclosures for either of the authors.
Department of Neuroscience/Ophthalmology, University Hospital, Uppsala University, Uppsala 75185, Sweden
* Corresponding authors.
E-mail addresses: gerd.holmstrom@neuro.uu.se; eva.larsson@neuro.uu.se

Clin Perinatol 40 (2013) 311–321
http://dx.doi.org/10.1016/j.clp.2013.02.008
0095-5108/13/$ – see front matter © 2013 Elsevier Inc. All rights reserved.

Table 1
Long-term ophthalmologic follow-up studies in prematurely born children who were screened prospectively for retinopathy of prematurity in the neonatal period

	Fledelius,[13,27,33,49] 1996	Darlow et al,[74] 1997	O'Connor et al,[25,50] 2002	Holmström, Larsson et al,[14,24,32,44,51,55,56,69] 2003-2006
Country	Denmark	New Zealand	United Kingdom	Sweden
Inclusion criteria	BW <2000 g GA <26 wk	BW <1500 g	BW <1701 g	BW <1501 g
Born	1982–1984	1986	1985–1987	1988–1990
Age at follow-up (y)	7–10	7–8	10–12	10
Number	88	274	254	216
Percentage of initial surviving cohort (%)	48	92	53	87
Comparison with control group	Previous control group	Previous control group	169	217
ROP	32%	21%	50%	39%
ROP, stages 3–5		4.4%	3.9%	19%
Treated	0	0	0	12%
Visual impairment	<20/200 4.1%	<20/200 2.9% <20/50 8%	<20/40 3.5%	<20/200 1.4% <20/60 1.9%
Strabismus	18%	22%	19%	16%
Myopia	<0D 13%	<0D 14%–21%	<0D 22% <–3D 4.7%	<0D 15% <–3D 3.8%
Hypermetropia		>+1D 18%	>+3D 9.2%	>+3D 4.2%
Astigmatism	≥1D 16%	≥1D 11%		≥1D 21%
Anisometropia	≥2D 6%			≥1D 8.9% ≥2D 5.2%

Abbreviations: BW, birth weight; D, diopter; GA, gestational age.

(CRYO-ROP) study and the Early Treatment for Retinopathy of Prematurity (ETROP) study.[5,6] Furthermore, Connolly and colleagues[7] compared the results of cryotreatment and laser treatment at the age of 10 years. The long-term outcome and effects of the recently introduced anti–vascular endothelial growth factor (VEGF) treatment are not yet known.

The aim of this article is to discuss the long-term outcome of ROP with respect to various visual and ophthalmologic aspects.

VISUAL ACUITY

Visual impairment and blindness in prematurely born children may be caused by retinal or cerebral abnormalities, or a combination of the two. Several studies claim that cerebral damage is becoming the most important cause.[8,9]

It has been suspected that the increasing survival of a new population of extremely prematurely born infants takes place at the expense of increased neurodevelopmental impairments, including visual impairment. Reassuringly, however, this does not seem to be the case in studies from Finland,[10] Great Britain,[11] Norway,[12] and Sweden (Fredrik Serenius, personal communication, 2012), which show similar prevalences (1%–2%) of blindness in extremely preterm children as in previous population-based studies of less preterm populations.[13,14]

Developing and improving treatment options and treatment criteria for ROP are continuously changing the visual outcome. In the CRYO-ROP study, 44% of cryo-treated children at a defined threshold disease were visually impaired ($\leq$20/200) at 10 years.[5] In the 1990s laser therapy was introduced, and in 2002 Ng and colleagues[15] compared the visual outcome in eyes treated with cryotherapy and laser, and reported better visual outcome in the latter. New criteria have since been introduced, showing that earlier treatment results in superior visual outcome for type 1 ROP at 6-year follow-up, compared with conventional treatment at threshold disease.[6,16] Today, laser therapy is the treatment of choice with regression of ROP in the majority of cases.[17,18]

As expected, in more advanced stages of ROP the visual outcome is worse. Hence, the CRYO-ROP study reveals a high proportion (94%) of unfavorable visual acuity in eyes with Zone I ROP.[5] Furthermore, despite treatment for aggressive posterior ROP (AP-ROP), a substantial proportion of eyes develop retinal detachments, most probably leading to very poor vision, if any.[18,19] Anti-VEGF treatment may improve structural and visual outcome of AP-ROP, but the systemic and ophthalmic long-term effects are still unknown.[20]

Lens-sparing vitrectomy for ROP stage 4A has shown positive results.[6,21] Disappointingly, the visual outcome after surgery for retinal detachment in stages 4B and 5 is usually very poor. In the study by Ng and colleagues,[15] none of the eyes with stages 4B and 5 had light perception, regardless of previous cryotreatment or laser treatment. Only 1 of the 9 eyes with stage 5 ROP in the ETROP study that were operated on with vitrectomy, with or without scleral buckling, had light perception.[22]

Various degrees of reduced visual acuities have been described in children with a history of ROP. As already described, eyes with the most severe stages of ROP are at the highest risk of visual impairment. Slightly reduced or subnormal visual acuity, however, is a common feature in eyes with a history of mild ROP and also in eyes without ROP, despite any obvious cerebral damage.[8,14] Minor retinal and/or cerebral factors have been suggested as possible causes of such subnormal vision.

Finally, it should be mentioned that visual perceptual deficits, including problems with recognition, orientation, depth perception, perception of movement, and simultaneous perception, are becoming common in prematurely born children and may significantly affect their daily life.[23] However, this issue is beyond the scope of this article, which mainly focuses on the effects of ROP.

REFRACTION

Prematurely born children have a higher prevalence of refractive errors than do children born at term.[24,25] In most studies, refraction is measured in cycloplegia, but the definitions of myopia and hypermetropia vary. Before term the eye is probably myopic, whereas at term the refraction has changed to hypermetropia.[26,27] During growth, refraction continuously changes toward emmetropia,[28] but the normal process of emmetropization may be altered, resulting in refractive errors. A disturbance in ocular growth and the development of the eye has been suggested in preterm children. This disturbance is primarily caused by changes in the anterior segment and axial length of the eye, such as steeper corneal curvature, shallow anterior chamber and thicker lens, and too short or too long an axial length.[29,30]

Various types of refractive errors have been described in prematurely born children. In particular, a high prevalence of myopia has been associated with preterm birth, including 3 major types[31]: first, a transient myopia that disappears within the first or second year of life[32]; second, myopia without previous ROP, myopia of prematurity (MOP)[24,33]; and third, myopia induced by severe ROP.[34–36] In the CRYO-ROP study, eyes with treated and untreated threshold ROP were compared and showed the same prevalence of myopia, indicating that severe ROP itself and not the treatment per se was the cause of myopia.[34] Later studies have indicated less myopia in treated eyes after laser treatment.[7] There are also small studies showing that eyes treated with lens-sparing vitrectomy have less myopia than those treated with laser alone.[37] The effect of anti-VEGF injections on refraction of the eye is as yet unknown. A small study of 18 eyes injected with bevacizumab revealed myopia at 5 years of age.[38] However, it could not be concluded whether the myopia was induced by the severe ROP or by the treatment itself.

The effect of the timing of treatment (early or late) on refractive outcome has also been investigated in the American ETROP study. The investigators stated that earlier treatment did not influence the development of refractive errors.[35] In a long-term Swedish population-based study of 10-year-old prematurely born children,[24] significant refractive errors, defined as spherical equivalent -1 diopter (D) or less than $+3$D and/or astigmatism of at least 1D and/or anisometropia of at least 1 D, were found in 30% of the children, compared with 8% in full-term children of the same age. The children with severe treated ROP had the highest prevalence (64%) of refractive errors, but no difference was found between those with a history of mild ROP and those without ROP. In addition, there was a higher prevalence of refractive errors in the children with no ROP (26%) than in those born at full term (8%), thus indicating that prematurity itself may affect emmetropization. Finally, regarding scleral buckling surgery, a risk of development of high myopia, anisometropia, and amblyopia should also be mentioned.[39]

VISUAL FIELDS

Peripheral ablation of the retina in the treatment of ROP is believed to constrict the visual field (VF).[40] The CRYO-ROP study, however, compared peripheral VF in eyes with treated and untreated threshold ROP, but could only find minor differences, indicating that severe ROP and the treatment itself both affect the VF.[41] A limited reduction in VF has also been reported in eyes treated with laser therapy.[42] The earlier treatment, introduced in the ETROP study, did not seem to further constrict the peripheral

VFs.[43] Finally, in a study by Larsson and colleagues[44] at 10 years of age, VFs in prematurely born children with various stages of ROP were compared with those of full-term children. The peripheral VF in cryotreated eyes was slightly constricted, whereas eyes with mild ROP or no ROP did not differ from the eyes of the full-term children. Within the central VF, inside 30° a reduced sensitivity was found in the whole group of prematurely born children, without any further reduction in the treated eyes. It should be emphasized that neurologic deficits in the prematurely born children, such as periventricular leukomalacia, may also affect the VF.[45]

STRABISMUS

Prematurity is an important risk factor for strabismus,[46] which has been confirmed in population-based studies comparing prematurely born children with full-term controls up to puberty and adolescence.[47,48] In follow-up studies at 10 to 12 years of age, 16% to 20% of prematurely born children had manifest strabismus, compared with around 3% of the normal population.[49–51] ROP is significantly correlated with strabismus, as are various neurologic abnormalities.[49–51] Furthermore, increasing stages of ROP increase the prevalence of strabismus, illustrated by the fact that 36% of children with previously cryotreated eyes had strabismus at 10 years of age,[51] and 44% of the children in the ETROP study had strabismus at 6 years of age.[52] Whether the increased risk of strabismus is caused by retinal sequelae, refractive errors, anisometropia, abnormal emmetropization, or a combination of these factors, can only be speculated upon.

It is interesting that the proportion of exotropia seems to be higher in prematurely born children than in the normal population, which has been attributed to a higher prevalence of neurologic problems in this group of children.[50,51] The natural course of strabismus up to 10 years was investigated in a population-based study, revealing that one-third of the children had an onset after 3.5 years, a finding that should be emphasized to parents.[51]

As a consequence of the increased prevalence of strabismus, stereopsis is also reduced in prematurely born children.[50,51] Furthermore, children without manifest strabismus are also reported to have reduced levels of stereopsis,[50,51] probably attributable to neurologic defects.

ACCOMMODATION AND CONVERGENCE

Accommodation and convergence have been assessed in only a few studies of prematurely born children.[53–55] Neither Dowdeswell and colleagues[53] nor Lindqvist and colleagues[54] found any impaired convergence, and the latter found no reduction in accommodation in preterm children. In these studies, however, the children were not screened for ROP in the neonatal period. In a study by Larsson and colleagues,[55] there was a small reduction of both accommodative amplitude and impaired convergence in prematurely born children when compared with full-term children, but no correlations with ROP were found.

CONTRAST SENSITIVITY

Contrast sensitivity (CS) is an important part of visual function and is essential for daily life. It is dependent on optical conditions, retinal function, and the posterior visual pathways, all of which may be affected in prematurely born children. Several studies have shown decreased CS in prematurely born children in comparison with those born at term.[25,54,56] In 2 long-term population-based studies, no difference was found between eyes without ROP and those with mild ROP.[25,56] A reduction of CS in eyes with treated ROP was found in the CRYO-ROP study, as well as in the study by Larsson and colleagues[56,57] However, in the CRYO-ROP study, the eyes with treated threshold ROP had better CS than eyes with untreated threshold ROP, thus supporting the beneficial effect of treatment.[57] As suspected, neurologic abnormalities affect CS, which was confirmed in a study by Fazzi and colleagues,[58] who found reduced CS in children with cerebral visual impairment. In preterm children, however, severe cryo-treated ROP, rather than neurologic complications, has been the main risk factor for reduced CS.[56]

RETINAL FUNCTION AND MORPHOLOGY

Retinal anatomy, morphology, and function in prematurely born children have been reported by various groups, up to teen age. Retinal abnormalities, such as pigmentary changes, degenerations, macular dragging/heterotopia, retinal folds, and detachments, are described in untreated as well as eyes treated for ROP.[59,60] In the 10-year follow-up of the CRYO-ROP study, 19% of the treated eyes had macular ectopia, partial retinal detachment, or a retinal fold not including macula, and 26% had partial or total retinal detachments.[5] In a 15-year follow-up, a further increase in the unfavorable structural outcome had occurred, and new posterior pole abnormalities and detachments were reported in some eyes.[61] Various retinal abnormalities, including late detachments, in both treated and untreated eyes, were also described in other studies, indicating that ROP seems to indeed be a lifelong disease.[3,15,62]

Two studies on retinal morphology with optical coherence tomography in prematurely born children up to 14 to 16 years of age have recently been performed.[63,64] These studies revealed thicker maculae and thinner retinal nerve-fiber layer, with the highest risk among those with the most severe ROP.[65] Åkerblom and colleagues[63] also found thicker maculae in preterm infants without ROP when compared with children born at term, with a correlation to the degree of prematurity per se. Moreover, electroretinographic studies on prematurely born children and full-term controls indicate abnormalities in photoreceptor functions in both rods and cones, again related to severity of ROP.[66,67] Only long-term follow-up studies will reveal the impact of these findings on future visual functions. Recently, Fledelius and Jensen[3] reported on insidious visual loss in 31 eyes of prematurely born adults up to 39 years of age. Some of the eyes had been treated for ROP, whereas others had not. The investigators speculate that the cause could be some kind of involutive retinal abnormality, possibly in combination with an aging retina. Future follow-up studies of prematurely born adults may reveal whether this is only the tip of an iceberg.

FOLLOW-UP ROUTINES AND GUIDELINES

As illustrated in this and previous articles, prematurely born children have an increased risk of various ophthalmic and visual dysfunctions and abnormalities, in particular those children with a history of severe and treatment-requiring ROP and those with severe cerebral sequelae. However, children without ROP or with mild ROP have an increased risk of problems, although they may seem subtle. In their long-term follow-ups at 10 to 12 years of age, Stephenson and colleagues[68] and Holmström and Larsson[69] reported abnormalities in 50% and 25% of the children, respectively, depending on definitions of "visual abnormalities." Some of the defects may indeed be subtle, but taken together they may affect the daily lives of these children and adults, particularly those with other sequelae, such as neurologic and visual perceptual deficiencies. Several studies have reported associations between various visual dysfunctions and school problems, supporting this opinion.[47,48,68,69]

The question of long-term ophthalmic follow-up guidelines is difficult, but important and unavoidable. Should all prematurely born children be followed up or should we focus on certain risk groups, and, in that case, which? Another question is when such follow-ups should be performed. Today there is certainly agreement on the need to follow children with treatment-requiring ROP and severe neurologic problems, but there is still no consensus regarding children with no ROP or with mild ROP. Recommendations regarding the latter groups also depend on available national health resources and organization. American guidelines state that ophthalmologic follow-up is indicated in children with ROP within 4 to 6 months after discharge, regardless of severity,[70] whereas others have recommended follow-up of all children at 2.5 years[69,71] and at school age.[71] It has also been proposed that national visual acuity tests at 4 to 5 years may pick up visual problems in this group.[72,73]

Regardless of guidelines for follow-up, it is important to continuously evaluate and modify such programs. There is also a need to provide information regarding visual dysfunction to parents, schools, and society as a whole. Extremely preterm children are today growing up with unknown long-term consequences for their visual functions.[62] We are therefore obliged to follow their outcome and support this new and surviving group of increasingly immature infants.

REFERENCES

1. Gilbert C. Changing challenges in the control of blindness in children. Eye 2007; 21:1338–43.
2. van Sorge AJ, Termote JU, de Vries MJ, et al. The incidence of visual impairment due to retinopathy of prematurity (ROP) and concomitant disabilities in the Netherlands: a 30 year overview. Br J Ophthalmol 2011;95:937–41.
3. Fledelius HC, Jensen H. Late subsequent ocular morbidity in retinopathy of prematurity patients, with emphasis on visual loss caused by insidious 'involutive' pathology: an observational series. Acta Ophthalmol 2011;89:316–23.
4. Smith BT, Tasman WS. Retinopathy of prematurity: late complications in the baby boomer generation (1946-1964). Trans Am Ophthalmol Soc 2005;103:225–34.
5. Cryotherapy for Retinopathy of Prematurity Cooperative Group. Multicenter trial of cryotherapy for retinopathy of prematurity: ophthalmological outcomes at 10 years. Arch Ophthalmol 2001;119:1110–8.
6. Early Treatment for Retinopathy of Prematurity Cooperative Group. Final visual acuity results in the early treatment for retinopathy of prematurity study. Arch Ophthalmol 2010;128:663–71.
7. Connolly BP, Ng EY, McNamara JA, et al. A comparison of laser photocoagulation with cryotherapy for threshold retinopathy of prematurity at 10 years of age. Ophthalmology 2002;109:936–41.
8. Slidsborg C, Bangsgaard R, Fledelius HC, et al. Cerebral damage may be the primary risk factor for visual impairment in preschool children born extremely premature. Arch Ophthalmol 2012;130(11):1410–7.
9. Rahi JS, Cable N, on behalf of the British Childhood Visual Impairment Study Group (BCVISG). Severe visual impairment and blindness in children in the UK. Lancet 2003;362:1359–65.
10. Tommiska V, Heinonen K, Kero P, et al. A national two year follow up study of extremely low birthweight infants born in 1996-1997. Arch Dis Child Fetal Neonatal Ed 2003;88:F29–35.

11. Wood NS, Marlow N, Costeloe K, et al. Neurologic and developmental disability after extremely preterm birth. EPICure Study Group. N Engl J Med 2000;343: 378–84.

12. Leversen KT, Sommerfelt K, Rønnestad A, et al. Prediction of neurodevelopmental and sensory outcome at 5 years in Norwegian children born extremely preterm. Pediatrics 2011;127:e630–8.

13. Fledelius HC. Pre-term delivery and subsequent ocular development. A 7-10 year follow-up of children screened 1982-84 for ROP. 1) Visual function, slit-lamp findings, and fundus appearance. Acta Ophthalmol Scand 1996;74: 288–93.

14. Larsson E, Rydberg A, Holmström G. A population-based study on the visual outcome in 10-year-old preterm and full-term children. Arch Ophthalmol 2005; 123:825–32.

15. Ng EY, Connolly BP, McNamara JA, et al. A comparison of laser photocoagulation with cryotherapy for threshold retinopathy of prematurity at 10 years: part 1. Visual function and structural outcome. Ophthalmology 2002;109:928–34.

16. Early Treatment for Retinopathy of Prematurity Cooperative Group. Revised indications for the treatment of retinopathy of prematurity: results of the early treatment for retinopathy of prematurity randomized trial. Arch Ophthalmol 2003;121: 1684–96.

17. Austeng D, Källen KB, Ewald UW, et al. Treatment for retinopathy of prematurity in infants born before 27 weeks of gestation in Sweden. Br J Ophthalmol 2010; 94:1136–9.

18. Gunn DJ, Cartwright DW, Yuen SA, et al. Treatment of retinopathy of prematurity in extremely premature infants over an 18 year period. Clin Experiment Ophthalmol 2013;41(2):159–66.

19. Sanghi G, Dogra MR, Katoch D, et al. Aggressive posterior retinopathy of prematurity: risk factors for retinal detachment despite confluent laser photocoagulation. Am J Ophthalmol 2013;155(1):159–164.e2.

20. Mintz-Hittner HA, Kennedy KA, Chuang AZ, BEAT-ROP Cooperative Group. Efficacy of intravitreal bevacizumab for stage 3+ retinopathy of prematurity. N Engl J Med 2011;364(7):603–15.

21. Prenner JL, Capone A Jr, Trese MT. Visual outcomes after lens-sparing vitrectomy for stage 4A retinopathy of prematurity. Ophthalmology 2004;111:2271–3.

22. Repka MX, Tung B, Good WV, et al. Outcome of eyes developing retinal detachment during the early treatment for retinopathy of prematurity study. Arch Ophthalmol 2011;129:1175–9.

23. Dutton G, Ballantyne J, Boyd G, et al. Cortical visual dysfunction in children. A clinical study. Eye 1996;10:302–9.

24. Larsson E, Rydberg A, Holmström G. A population-based study of the refractive outcome in 10-year-old preterm and full-term children. Arch Ophthalmol 2003; 121:1430–6.

25. O'Connor AR, Stephenson T, Johnson A, et al. Long-term ophthalmic outcome of low birth weight children with and without retinopathy of prematurity. Pediatrics 2002;109:12–8.

26. Gordon RA, Donzis PB. Refractive development of the human eye. Arch Ophthalmol 1985;103:785–9.

27. Fledelius HC. Pre-term delivery and growth of the eye. An oculometric study of eye size around term-time. Acta Ophthalmol Suppl 1992;(204):10–5.

28. Mayer DL, Hansen RM, Moore BD, et al. Cycloplegic refraction in healthy children aged 1 through 48 months. Arch Ophthalmol 2001;119:1625–8.

29. Fledelius HC. Pre-term delivery and subsequent ocular development. A 7-10 year follow-up of children screened 1982-84 for ROP. 4) Ocularmetric and other metric considerations. Acta Ophthalmol 1996;74:301–5.

30. Chen TC, Tsai TH, Shih YF, et al. Long-term evaluation of refractive status and optical components in eyes of children born prematurely. Invest Ophthalmol Vis Sci 2010;51:6140–8.

31. Fielder AR, Quinn GE. Myopia of prematurity: nature, nurture, or disease? Br J Ophthalmol 1997;81:2–3.

32. Holmström G, Larsson E. Development of spherical equivalent refraction in prematurely-born children during the first 10 years of life—a population-based study. Arch Ophthalmol 2005;123:1404–11.

33. Fledelius HC. Pre-term delivery and subsequent ocular development. A 7-10 year follow-up of children screened 1982-84 for ROP. 3) Refraction. Myopia of prematurity. Acta Ophthalmol 1996;74:297–300.

34. Quinn GE, Dobson V, Siatkowski R, et al, Cryotherapy for Retinopathy of Prematurity Cooperative Group. Does cryotherapy affect refractive error? Results from the treated versus control eyes in the cryotherapy for retinopathy of prematurity trial. Ophthalmology 2001;108:343–7.

35. Quinn GE, Dobson V, Davitt BV, et al, on behalf of the Early Treatment for Retinopathy of Prematurity Cooperative Group. Progression of myopia and high myopia in the early treatment for retinopathy of prematurity study. Findings to 3 years of age. Ophthalmology 2008;115:1058–64.

36. O'Connor AR, Stephenson TJ, Johnson A, et al. Change in refractive state and eye size in children of birth weight less than 1701 g. Br J Ophthalmol 2006;90:456–60.

37. Carvounis PE, Poll J, Weikert MP, et al. Vitrectomy for retinopathy of prematurity. Arch Ophthalmol 2010;128:843–6.

38. Martínez-Castellanos MA, Schwartz S, Hernández-Rojas ML, et al. Long-term effect of antiangiogenic therapy for retinopathy of prematurity. Up to 5 years of follow-up. Retina 2013;33(2):329–38.

39. Chow DR, Ferrone PJ, Trese MT. Refractive changes associated with scleral buckling and division in retinopathy of prematurity. Arch Ophthalmol 1998;116:1446–8.

40. Takayama S, Tachibana H, Yamamoto M. Changes in the visual field after photocoagulation or cryotherapy in children with retinopathy of prematurity. J Pediatr Ophthalmol Strabismus 1991;28:96–100.

41. Cryotherapy for Retinopathy of Prematurity Cooperative Group. Effect of retinal ablative therapy for threshold retinopathy of prematurity: results of Goldmann perimetry at the age of 10 years. Arch Ophthalmol 2001;119:1120–5.

42. McLoone E, O'Keefe M, McLoone S, et al. Effect of diode laser ablative therapy for threshold retinopathy of prematurity on the visual field: results of Goldmann perimetry at a mean age of 11 years. J Pediatr Ophthalmol Strabismus 2007;44:170–3.

43. Early Treatment for Retinopathy of Prematurity Cooperative Group. Visual field extent at 6 years of age in children who had high-risk prethreshold retinopathy of prematurity. Arch Ophthalmol 2011;129:127–32.

44. Larsson E, Martin L, Holmström G. Peripheral and central visual fields in 11-year-old children who had been born prematurely and at term. J Pediatr Ophthalmol Strabismus 2004;41:39–45.

45. Dutton GN, Jacobson LK. Cerebral visual impairment in children. Semin Neonatol 2001;6:477–85.

46. Cotter SA, Varma R, Tarczy-Hornoch K, et al, Joint Writing Committee for the Multi-Ethnic Pediatric Eye Disease Study and the Baltimore Pediatric Eye Disease Study Groups. Risk factors associated with childhood strabismus: the multi-ethnic pediatric eye disease and Baltimore pediatric eye disease studies. Ophthalmology 2011;118:2251–61.

47. Hellgren K, Hellström A, Jacobson L, et al. Visual and cerebral sequelae of very low birth weight in adolescents. Arch Dis Child Fetal Neonatal Ed 2007;92: F259–64.

48. Lindqvist S, Vik T, Indredavik MS, et al. Eye movements and binocular function in low birthweight teenagers. Acta Ophthalmol 2008;86:265–74.

49. Fledelius HC. Pre-term delivery and subsequent ocular development. A 7-10 year follow-up of children screened 1982-84 for ROP. 2) Binocular function. Acta Ophthalmol Scand 1996;74:294–6.

50. O'Connor AR, Stephenson TJ, Johnson A, et al. Strabismus in children of birth weight less than 1701 g. Arch Ophthalmol 2002;120:767–73.

51. Holmström G, Rydberg A, Larsson E. Prevalence and development of strabismus in 10-year-old premature children: a population-based study. J Pediatr Ophthalmol Strabismus 2006;43:346–52.

52. VanderVeen DK, Bremer DL, Fellows RR, et al, Early Treatment for Retinopathy of Prematurity Cooperative Group. Prevalence and course of strabismus through age 6 years in participants of the Early Treatment for Retinopathy of Prematurity randomized trial. J AAPOS 2011;15:536–40.

53. Dowdeswell HJ, Slater AM, Broomhall J, et al. Visual deficits in children born at less than 32 weeks' gestation with and without major ocular pathology and cerebral damage. Br J Ophthalmol 1995;79:447–52.

54. Lindqvist S, Vik T, Indredavik MS, et al. Visual acuity, contrast sensitivity, peripheral vision and refraction in low birthweight teenagers. Acta Ophthalmol Scand 2007;85:157–64.

55. Larsson E, Rydberg A, Holmström G. Accommodation and convergence in 10-year-old prematurely born and full-term children—a population-based study. Strabismus 2012;20:127–32.

56. Larsson E, Rydberg A, Holmström G. Contrast sensitivity in 10-year-old preterm and full-term children—a population-based study. Br J Ophthalmol 2006;90: 87–90.

57. Cryotherapy for Retinopathy of Prematurity Cooperative Group. Contrast sensitivity at age 10 years in children who had threshold retinopathy of prematurity. Arch Ophthalmol 2001;119:1129–33.

58. Fazzi E, Signorini SG, La Piana R, et al. Neuro-ophthalmological disorders in cerebral palsy: ophthalmological, oculomotor, and visual aspects. Dev Med Child Neurol 2012;54:730–6.

59. International Committee for the Classification of the Late Stages of Retinopathy of Prematurity. An international classification of retinopathy of prematurity. II. The classification of retinal detachment. Arch Ophthalmol 1987;105:906–12.

60. Gallo JE, Holmström G, Kugelberg U, et al. Regressed retinopathy of prematurity and its sequelae in children aged 5-10 years. Br J Ophthalmol 1991;75: 527–31.

61. Palmer EA, Hardy RJ, Dobson V, et al, Cryotherapy for Retinopathy of Prematurity Cooperative Group. 15-year outcomes following threshold retinopathy of prematurity: final results from the multicenter trial of cryotherapy for retinopathy of prematurity. Arch Ophthalmol 2005;123:311–8.

62. Wheeler DT, Dobson V, Chiang MF, et al. Retinopathy of prematurity in infants weighing less than 500 grams at birth enrolled in the early treatment for retinopathy of prematurity study. Ophthalmology 2011;118:1145-51.

63. Åkerblom H, Larsson E, Eriksson U, et al. Central macular thickness is correlated with gestational age at birth in prematurely born children. Br J Ophthalmol 2011;95:799-803.

64. Wu WC, Lin RI, Shih CP, et al. Visual acuity, optical components, and macular abnormalities in patients with a history of retinopathy of prematurity. Ophthalmology 2012;119:1907-16.

65. Åkerblom H, Holmström G, Eriksson U, et al. Retinal nerve fibre layer thickness in school-aged prematurely-born children compared to children born at term. Br J Ophthalmol 2012;96:956-60.

66. Fulton AB, Hansen RM, Petersen RA, et al. The rod receptors in retinopathy of prematurity: an electroretinographic study. Arch Ophthalmol 2001;119:499-505.

67. Fulton AB, Hansen RM, Moskowitz A. The cone electroretinogram in retinopathy of prematurity. Invest Ophthalmol Vis Sci 2008;49:814-9.

68. Stephenson T, Wright S, O'Connor A, et al. Children born weighing less than 1701 g: visual and cognitive outcomes at 11-14 years. Arch Dis Child Fetal Neonatal Ed 2007;92:F265-70.

69. Holmström G, Larsson E. Long-term follow-up of visual functions in prematurely born children—a prospective population-based study up to 10 years of age. J AAPOS 2008;12:157-62.

70. American Academy of Pediatrics, the American Association of Pediatric Ophthalmology and Strabismus and the American Academy of Ophthalmology. Screening Examination of Premature Infants for Retinopathy of Prematurity. A joint statement by the American Academy of Pediatrics, the American Association of Pediatric Ophthalmology and Strabismus and the American Academy of Ophthalmology. Pediatrics 2013;131:189-95.

71. Schalij-Delfos NE, de Graaf ME, Treffers WF, et al. Long term follow up of premature infants: detection of strabismus, amblyopia, and refractive errors. Br J Ophthalmol 2000;84:963-7.

72. O'Connor AR, Stewart CE, Singh J, et al. Do infants of birth weight less than 1500 g require additional long term ophthalmic follow up? Br J Ophthalmol 2006;90:451-5.

73. Hård AL, Hellström A. Ophthalmological follow-up at 2 years of age of all children previously screened for retinopathy of prematurity: is it worthwhile? Acta Ophthalmol Scand 2006;84:631-5.

74. Darlow BA, Clemett RC, Horwood LJ, et al. Prospective study of New Zeeland infants with birth weight less than 1500 g and screened for retinopathy of prematurity: visual outcome at age 7-8 years. Br J Ophthalmol 1997;81:935-40.

Lessons in Retinopathy of Prematurity from Shanghai

Graham E. Quinn, MD, MSCE[a],*,
Alistair R. Fielder, FRCP, FRCS, FRCOphth[b],
Rajvardhan Azad, MBBS, MD, FRCSed[c], Peiquan Zhao, MD[d]

KEYWORDS

- Retinopathy of prematurity • Postnatal weight gain • Anti-VEGF agents
- World ROP Congress

KEY POINTS

- There is no one-size-fits-all guideline for retinopathy of prematurity (ROP) screening because the birth weight and gestational age characteristics of babies at risk of sight-threatening ROP differ between countries and even between neonatal intensive care units within one city.
- The diversity in the risk of developing ROP between centers is likely due to differing standards of neonatal care; the role of the neonatal team, especially the nurse, is critical in ensuring that improvements will have an immediate impact on reducing much sight-threatening ROP.
- Fluorescein angiography and optical coherence tomography allow improved visualization of the retina in vivo, the latter at a microscopic level.
- Innovative methods of identifying the baby at risk of severe ROP have been recently developed, including those based on postnatal weight gain that aim to reduce the number of ophthalmic examinations. Digital imaging has provided the opportunity for telemedicine and the automated analysis of the retinal image.
- There is a flurry of activity in the use of anti–vascular endothelial growth factor agents to treat ROP. Although there is agreement that acute ROP does respond to these drugs, there is no consensus on which eyes benefit functionally and what systemic adverse effects may occur. There is a pressing need to determine the safe dose for the eye and the baby.

In these days when interdisciplinary basic research and multiprofessional clinical research and practice are at the heart of progress, one wonders if it makes sense to hold a world congress on a single eye condition. After all, though it may attract some of the major researchers in the field, it has limitations when it comes to attracting

[a] Division of Ophthalmology, University of Pennsylvania, The Children's Hospital of Philadelphia, Wood Center, 1st Floor, Philadelphia, PA 19104, USA; [b] Department of Optometry & Visual Science, City University, Northampton Square, London EC1V 0HB, UK; [c] Dr. R.P. Centre for Ophthalmic Sciences, All India Institute of Medical Sciences, Ansari Nagar, New Delhi 110 029, India; [d] Xinhua Hospital, School of Medicine, Shanghai Jiao Tong University, 1665 Kong Jiang Road, Shanghai 200092, China
* Corresponding author.
E-mail address: QUINN@email.chop.edu

Clin Perinatol 40 (2013) 323–327
http://dx.doi.org/10.1016/j.clp.2013.02.009
0095-5108/13/$ – see front matter © 2013 Elsevier Inc. All rights reserved.

the attendance and participation of clinicians and scientists who want more than one topic from a conference. So what are the benefits of holding a world congress solely for retinopathy of prematurity (ROP), and do they outweigh the possible limitations?

There have been great advances in our understanding of the fundamental pathogenesis of ROP, its risk factors, and how ROP should be identified and treated. As a result of these improvements, blindness has been reduced in many countries, but the situation is patchy, and in many countries ROP remains a major cause of visual disability in childhood. In addition, in those countries which have a relatively low incidence of ROP blindness, this has only been achieved by a very high consumption of health resources, making ROP screening relatively effective but far from efficient. One of main the purposes of the recent World ROP Congress, held in October 2012, was to gather together basic scientists, ophthalmologists, nurses, and neonatologists, individuals who would not normally be in the same room, to explore the nature of variations across the world and work toward the elimination ROP blindness. World ROP Congresses have been held in a region of the world where there is local enthusiasm for the conference and yet where the need is great, so serving to raise the profile of ROP blindness in that area. Accordingly, the first World ROP Congress was held in Vilnius, Lithuania in 2006, with the second meeting being in Delhi in 2009; and so to the World ROP Congress, Shanghai 2012.

Several presentations at the 2012 Congress addressed the important issue of defining the birth weight (BW) and gestational age (GA) characteristics of the baby at risk of ROP. Sweden is the first, and so far the only country, to establish a national ROP registry, which now includes more than 4000 babies, 96% of Swedish babies of less than 32 weeks GA. No infant with GA more than 28 weeks required treatment, although a few (n = 9) babies with a greater GA developed stage 3, not requiring treatment. However, the situation in Sweden is not representative of all other countries. Presentations from Brazil, China, Egypt, India, Kazakhstan, Mexico, and Russia told a different story, and all reported ROP requiring treatment in larger and more mature babies, in some instances in babies more than 2000 g BW and more than 34 weeks GA. A presentation from Brazil made the important point that, reflecting the standards of neonatal care, the ROP risk, in terms of GA and BW, for babies can vary not only between countries but also between individual neonatal intensive care units within one city, with the consequence that screening inclusion criteria could be narrower in the "better" units. The relatively recently described aggressive posterior ROP (AP-ROP) is the most serious form of ROP and the most difficult to treat, and its causation is poorly understood. AP-ROP is rare in the high-income countries such as the United Kingdom, accounting for less than 1% of ROP, and is exclusive to the most premature babies. Several presentations, mainly from India, reported AP-ROP to occur in larger babies even heavier than 2000 g BW and greater than 34 weeks GA. Evidence was presented that, in larger babies at least, the standard of neonatal care is likely the most important causative factor for AP-ROP, notably the unregulated or poorly regulated use of supplemental oxygen.

Presentations from New Zealand, Argentina, and Mexico highlighted the importance of neonatal teamwork in reducing ROP, with the need for high-quality nurse training and achievement of adequate nurse/baby ratios. Monitoring equipment needs to be available and used appropriately. The neonatal team, especially the nurse, is essential in the maintenance the baby's stability, to prevent and treat infection and also to alleviate pain. Involvement of the parents in their baby's care very early empowers parents and promotes attendance at follow-up appointments. A powerful message emerged from these presentations: that the standard of neonatal care is critical with respect to the risk of ROP, and that this is one area where improvements will have an immediate impact and prevent much sight-threatening ROP.

Screening (or more properly the diagnostic examination for the detection of ROP) was the subject of several presentations that highlighted how the population at risk differs across the world. Sweden, at the high end of the excellence spectrum in terms of neonatal care, has been able to reduce its inclusion criteria for screening from less than 32 weeks GA to less than 31 weeks GA, but has added the recommendation that neonatologists refer for screening more mature preterm babies who are "generally ill or have several comorbidities." In China, on the other hand, screening is recommended for babies lighter than 2000 g and for heavier babies if the baby is considered to have a high risk for ROP, whereas in Mexico it is recommended that babies of less than 36 weeks GA with 5 or more days of ventilation are screened. With advances in neonatal management, screening requirements will inevitably need to be updated from time to time. At present there is no single screening guideline that fits all situations, and clearly there is some way to go in guideline development. One thought emerges from learning the experiences from different countries: will it be possible to define inclusion criteria that would identify the majority of babies at risk of ROP? If this can be achieved, will it then be feasible to separately determine the risk factors that require larger and more mature babies to be screened? If so, this would reduce the number of babies that need to be examined.

Screening remains one of the major topics in the ROP world in high-, medium-, and low-income countries, and for many reasons. Workshops in Latin America have been shown to be an excellent model whereby local challenges have been addressed, akin to the ROP roadshows held in the United Kingdom several years ago. The aim of screening is to lead to the timely identification of the eye requiring treatment while avoiding unnecessary examinations, so it needs to be both effective and efficient. ROP screening consumes considerable health resources in terms of time and expertise. For instance, the examination requires highly specialist ophthalmic skills, which in some countries are not readily available for several reasons, and it takes about 40 examinations[1] to identify one baby requiring treatment; both of these factors should act as a stimulus for innovation in screening. There were several presentations in Shanghai addressing this issue, which fell into 2 major categories: first, screening by avoiding the eye examination and second, examination using digital imaging. Research in Sweden[2] first demonstrated that an algorithm (WINROP) based on postnatal weight gain, measured weekly, identifies babies at high risk of developing severe ROP and so predicts ROP requiring treatment. WINROP was first tested in Sweden and subsequently on more diverse populations in the United States and Latin America. In general, it has a high sensitivity and negative predictive value, but lower specificity for predicting severe ROP. Other algorithms have since been developed, notably CHOP ROP[3] from Philadelphia. All produce similar results and show promise in reducing the need for ophthalmic screening examinations. To date, all postnatal weight gain algorithms have been used in a research setting, but this is definitely a case of "watch this space" for their introduction into routine clinical practice, although it must be anticipated that they are unlikely to be of value in the heavier, more mature baby in whom ROP progression is compressed.

The diagnosis of ROP is entirely visual, but qualitative, and is well known to be prone to error. One might have expected the advent of digital imaging in the 1990s to be an answer to the ophthalmologist's prayer to address many of the challenges of screening, because it permitted for the first time the retinal findings to be recorded and, if need be, electronically transmitted to remote sites: the opportunity for telemedicine. It was not to be so, in part due to reluctance by the ophthalmic community to accept the validity of digital imaging for recording the ROP lesion (and its expense). In addition, the concept of telemedicine using electronic transmission in middle-income countries, where it was most needed, was not fully accepted. So it was exciting to hear at last, in 2012 in Shanghai, of exciting and innovative telemedicine programs and studies in India and the United States, all reporting the success of telemedicine in identifying severe ROP by a centralized expert who evaluated images obtained remotely by a trained technician. A major multicenter study (eROP) is now under way in the United States. Digital imaging is also of value in monitoring eye treatment.

Digital imaging has opened many new opportunities, and already further developments are under way such as enhancement of the retinal image and automated quantitative analysis of retinal vessels which, it is hoped, will lead to a quantitative analysis of plus disease, a current indication for treatment. Another anticipated development is the automated analysis of retinal vessels, which will permit the eye that needs an examination by an ophthalmologist to be differentiated from the eye with no or mild ROP.

Moving away from screening, there were several presentations on 2 further imaging technologies that show promise: fluorescein angiography and optical coherence tomography (OCT). Both have been routinely and frequently used for years to study retinal disease in adults, but, for several technical reasons, only recently has their use been possible on the neonatal eye. Neither technology is applicable to everyday routine use, but fluorescein angiography, albeit not entirely noninvasive, has clearly demonstrated oxygen-induced retraction of formed retinal vessels that could not otherwise be visualized, and has provided invaluable insight into ROP pathogenesis especially with respect to AP-ROP. This characteristic was demonstrated in experimental animals in the 1950s,[4,5] but was not confirmed in the human until 2012.[6] OCT, with presentations from Russia, the United States, and India, allows a cross-sectional in vivo, as distinct from postmortem, microscopic examination of the central retina. Not yet widely in use, this technology is already providing new insights at a cellular and subcellular level into normal retinal development, the acute ROP process, and its long-term sequelae.

Although laser is currently the standard treatment for severe acute-phase ROP, without doubt the "hot topic" of the Congress was the use of anti–vascular endothelial growth factor (anti-VEGF) agents as a treatment modality. How is it possible that an off-label treatment came to be used worldwide without a research evidence base concerning its use in neonates? The reason, of course, lies in its use in adults in the treatment of age-related macular degeneration and other retinal conditions, for which bevacizumab (Avastin), along with other anti-VEGF agents, has been exceptionally successful and has generated a revolution in the world of ophthalmology. At the Shanghai ROP World Congress there were many presentations from several countries—China, India, Japan, Mexico, Taiwan, United States, and Vietnam—all reporting favorable structural outcomes with this treatment, mostly with bevacizumab, used as a monotherapy or in combination with laser. To date there has been only one randomized controlled trial using anti-VEGF agents, namely the BEAT ROP study[7] from Houston, Texas, which used bevacizumab. This study, not without controversy particularly with respect to its methodology, reported that benefit was restricted to eyes with ROP only in Zone I. While all presentations were encouraging regarding the use of anti-VEGF treatment in acute-phase ROP at this juncture, there is no clear and precise message about which eyes may or may not benefit from this treatment. As with laser, timing may be critical, so that treatment should be administered when acute-phase ROP is active and before the fibrotic process has yet to commence. Treatment when fibrosis/gliosis has commenced carries a risk of hastening progression to retinal detachment. Some presentations reported a high success rate with only one dose of anti-VEGF, whereas others reported the presence of vascular shunts a few weeks after treatment, sometimes leading to retinal detachment.[8] Whether these changes, occurring up to 60 to 70 weeks postmenstrual age and after seeming resolution, represent a true recurrence of the ROP or, as one presenter proposed, smoldering of the initial process, has yet to be clarified. An urgent priority is to determine which anti-VEGF agent is the best for use in the neonate, as well as what is the safe dose for the eye and the baby. Work from Japan confirmed reports from the literature that bevacizumab injected into the vitreous reaches the serum, and at 2 weeks after injection levels are still rising and serum VEGF levels are depressed. No adverse systemic effects have yet been identified, but a presentation from New Zealand drew the attention of participants that anti-VEGF agents act on vasculogenesis in many organs other than the eye; these include pulmonary alveolization, and development of the bones, heart, and kidney. VEGF is both neuroprotective and neurotropic. This presentation also reminded attendees of the difficulty in differentiating the possible effects of anti-VEGF agents from those attributable to preterm birth per se, and also its complications. As anti-VEGF agents are already being widely used, gaining an understanding of the optimum dose to inject into the eye, and its possible systemic effects, are the most urgent priorities. Clinical practice is far ahead of the evidence base, and this is not a healthy situation.

The third World ROP Congress held in Shanghai was a great success, and it was good to see that international collaborations have already built up from the previous 2 events. The participants learned about ROP from across the world: who it affects and its behavior, and in a way that would not be possible from the literature. Emerging technologies and treatments are set to have a major impact on ROP identification and treatment. Undoubtedly, in these exciting times the picture will have changed dramatically by the fourth World ROP Congress in Mexico in 3 years.

REFERENCES

1. Zin AA, Moreira ME, Bunce C, et al. Retinopathy of prematurity in 7 neonatal units in Rio de Janeiro: screening criteria and workload implications. Pediatrics 2010; 126:e410–7.
2. Wu C, Löfqvist C, Smith LE, et al, WINROP Consortium. Importance of early postnatal weight gain for normal retinal angiogenesis in very preterm infants: a multicenter study analyzing weight velocity deviations for the prediction of retinopathy of prematurity. Arch Ophthalmol 2012;130:992–9.
3. Binenbaum G, Ying GS, Quinn GE, et al. The CHOP postnatal weight gain, birth weight, and gestational age retinopathy of prematurity risk model. Arch Ophthalmol 2012;130:1560–5.
4. Ashton N. Oxygen and retinal blood vessels. Trans Ophthalmol Soc U K 1980; 100:359–62.
5. Patz A. Role of oxygen on immature retinal vessels. Invest Ophthalmol Vis Sci 1965;4:988–99.
6. Shah PK, Narendran V, Kalpan N. Aggressive posterior retinopathy of prematurity in large preterm babies in South India. Arch Dis Child Fetal Neonatal Ed 2012;97: F371–5.
7. Mintz-Hittner HA, Kennedy KA, Chuang AZ, BEAT-ROP Cooperative Group. Efficacy of intravitreal bevacizumab for stage 3+ retinopathy of prematurity. N Engl J Med 2011;364:603–15.
8. Hu J, Blair MP, Shapiro MJ, et al. Reactivation of retinopathy of prematurity after bevacizumab injection. Arch Ophthalmol 2012;130:1000–6.

Index

Note: Page numbers of article titles are in **boldface** type.

A

Accommodation, 315
Admission Booklet, for parents, 223
Aflibercept, 299
Angiogenesis
    in retinal development, 203, 207
    normal versus pathologic, 231
Animal models, of ROP, 204–209
ANZNN (Australian and New Zealand Neonatal Network) study, 186
Arachidonic acid, for retinal development, 209
A-scans, in OCT, 279
Australian and New Zealand Neonatal Network (ANZNN) study, 186
Automation, for ROP image analysis, 252–255

B

BEAT-ROP (Bevacizumab Eliminates the Angiogenic Threat of ROP) study, 186, 189, 299, 307, 326–327
Bevacizumab, 186, 189, 206, 299–308, 314
Bevacizumab Eliminates the Angiogenic Threat of ROP (BEAT-ROP) study, 186, 189, 299, 307, 326–327
Bioptigen OCT system, 274
Birth weight
    as issue at World Congress of 2012, **323–327**
    in screening criteria, 243–245, 249
Blindness, in ROP, incidence of, **185–200**
BLISS charity, 219
BOOST (Benefits of Oxygen Saturation Targeting) study, 232–236

C

CAIAR (Computer-Aided Image Analysis of the Retina), 253–254
Cameras, digital, 250–252
Canadian Neonatal Network study, 186
Canadian Oxygen Trial (COT), 234
CHOP ROP model, of Children's Hospital of Philadelphia, 264–266, 325
Classic retinopathy of prematurity, 244, 246
Clipping artifact, in OCT, 278
Color Doppler OCT, 282
Computer-Aided Image Analysis of the Retina (CAIAR), 253–254
Contrast sensitivity, 315–316
Convergence, 315

Clin Perinatol 40 (2013) 329–335
http://dx.doi.org/10.1016/S0095-5108(13)00046-8   perinatology.theclinics.com
0095-5108/13/$ – see front matter © 2013 Elsevier Inc. All rights reserved.

Moving?

Make sure your subscription moves with you!

To notify us of your new address, find your **Clinics Account Number** (located on your mailing label above your name), and contact customer service at:

Email: journalscustomerservice-usa@elsevier.com

800-654-2452 (subscribers in the U.S. & Canada)
314-447-8871 (subscribers outside of the U.S. & Canada)

Fax number: 314-447-8029

Elsevier Health Sciences Division
Subscription Customer Service
3251 Riverport Lane
Maryland Heights, MO 63043

*To ensure uninterrupted delivery of your subscription, please notify us at least 4 weeks in advance of move.

Printed and bound by CPI Group (UK) Ltd, Croydon, CR0 4YY

03/10/2024

01040440-0018